Releasing Arthritis:

The Seven Year Plan

Linda Frazer Fleming

PO Box 3175
Falls Church, VA 22043

Edited by Mary Abrams

Typography by Michael Leclair

Printed in USA by THE GOETZ PRINTING CO.

Cover Design by John Richard Fleming

Cover Photo by Tracy Rupp

Library of Congress Catalog Card Number: 89-92230

ISBN #1-877631-02-7

Dedication

You
On the Bottom
Too Weak to Lift Your Head
To You
Who Know That
Life
Hangs by a Thread
Hold On

Acknowledgments

I thank my husband, John Richard Fleming,
for his constant love and support.
I never knew that life
could be so sweet.

I thank my parents, brother, and sisters
for standing by me
when it would have been easier
to turn away.

As I celebrate my love for each of you,
I know
that I finally love myself.

Breezes

No more
stagnant air
standing still
Afraid.

Now,
Gently reaching breezes
Touch
The corners of my mind
With
Life.

Movement...
Waves of strength
Allow
No more waste.

A mind,
Finally clear,
Bending,
Savoring the breezes.

Swaying
With
Joy.

TABLE OF CONTENTS

FOREWORD

This is a book about recovering from illness, and more. It's also about learning how not to be ill. It was written to describe my experience in dealing with a specific disease, but I know that the path I took could have helped release any illness, mental or physical. The writing grew from my feeling that it was important to share my understanding of the healing potential within every human being. It is based on the belief that every human being deserves good health and that everyone has the power to heal, in every aspect of life.

There is little point in describing all the illnesses of my past, for I believe that my progressive recovery from rheumatoid arthritis also contains the essentials for healing other ailments I have had. Enough to say that from a very early age, my life was dominated by one major physical disaster after another, starting with an ulcer when I was seven, and moving on to rheumatoid arthritis at age 19.

As I began to write this book, I found myself reliving mentally the pain that I no longer felt physically. Writing, one of the biggest pleasures in my life, became a chore. On some level, I realized that I was reliving the pain because I still wasn't ready to let it go. I decided to honor my feelings of discomfort, but to continue working to see the past as a textbook, to be learned from and then set aside.

To my surprise, that decision, and the process of writing this book, opened another phase of my healing process. Each day before starting to write, I made it a habit to think about all the things I had learned over the years. I practiced feeling good about what I had accomplished, and telling myself that I could also be successful at learning whatever else I needed. As I persisted with that line of thinking, something wonderful happened. My dread of writing disappeared and feelings of amazement and joy at how far I've come took over. I began to look forward to sharing my life.

So often in the past I have picked up books like this to give to family or friends. I'd underline important parts and mail them off, proud that I was helping someone. The problem was that I neglected to learn anything from the books before I passed them along. It's true that Aunt Alice or your college roommate might find something very helpful in this book, but please don't just ship it out. First try to apply some of these ideas to yourself. Other people will learn more from the way you live your life than from what you suggest, ask, or tell them to do.

If reading this book helps you in any way, it was well worth the time it took me to commit to the process of change. Frankly, I had no idea that it would take seven years.

So where to start? At the beginning? That's a problem, because I can't really say where the beginning was. It seems logical to start by explaining that I tried every method of healing I heard or read about, every marginally plausible scheme friends suggested, every likely and unlikely cure that caught my eye, and then simply persevered until I gained the strength to search inside myself for the answers.

But perhaps I am moving too fast. Maybe the first thing I need to do is explain the suicide pact, or possibly move even further back in time. I'm still not sure where the story begins, but let's start with November 21, 1981.

I. A LOOK IN THE MIRROR

On November 21, 1981, I really looked at myself in the mirror for the first time in years, and I didn't like the person I saw looking back. The eyes facing me were surrounded by a 27-year-old atrophied body—a body that could perform only the simplest of tasks. I stood there wondering what had happened to the Linda I had once known—to the eyes that had once sparkled with hope for the future. I couldn't even imagine what I was about to put myself through.

The body I saw before me was a cruel reflection of the heart that it housed, a heart that beat with the dull ache of failure. I asked my vision to show me how to confront what had become of my life, but all that returned was a glare that pulsed with rage. Searching my face for any sign of hope or optimism, I was struck by the sight of my jaw, clamped tight in bitterness and pain.

As I felt a wall building between me and the woman in the mirror, I forced myself to be present for just a few more minutes. Hanging on to the sink, I opened my eyes for one more look.

This time, instead of seeing the body before me, my senses roared with the sound of my fragile life breaking into pieces, destroyed by mishandling. Imagining the longest and deepest breach, I knew that this overwhelming feeling represented my choice to turn from the task of deciding who I was. The strain of choosing a mindless existence over a committed one had finally taken its toll.

I never had allowed myself to express my feelings; crying was an unthinkable show of weakness. But the pain and immobility in my body had become a substitute for the tears I refused to shed and the life of joy that I refused to live. Refusal was no longer enough to keep me alive. My parched eyes and mouth begged me to find another way to live before it was too late to try.

Standing there, I heard a wail emerge from my throat so piercing that it scared me back into silence. It seemed to emerge from a space beyond my control. It didn't even resemble any sound I had ever heard at the movies. Shocked, I hobbled from the bathroom and busied myself in the bedroom, hoping my husband hadn't heard.

For days after that, I refused to meet my eyes in the mirror. Looking at my image brought up such feelings of hopelessness and guilt that I couldn't tolerate my reflection. But that first clear-eyed confrontation had somehow started the process of change.

II. HAPPY BIRTHDAY, LINDA

My 27th birthday, November 21, 1981, started with an unearthly scream. My husband and two cats shot to the ceiling; pillows flew across the room and lamps crashed to the floor. After scrambling for his glasses and glancing quickly around the room, my husband glared at me accusingly. The intruder he had hoped to blame for his rude awakening was nowhere to be seen.

Neither of us openly acknowledged the presence of an unwelcome guest in our house, present at my half-hearted invitation. Neither of us really recognized the part of me that wanted a better life, and that could no longer be ignored. My husband, no more comfortable with the intruding presence than I, never slept well in our bed again.

As for me, I had no conscious idea of what was happening. This incident, just one of a series, bolstered my fear that I was going crazy. The Linda I had always presented to the world had been a tightly controlled robot; this new behavior, unpredictable and terrifying, left me feeling as if someone else had taken control of my life and was running it without my consent.

A Declaration of War

That morning's scream was the first solid declaration of a war that had been waging inside me for two decades. On one side was the part of me that accepted the horror of my life as something totally under the control of others. There was another side, however, that kept charging back to assert that I did have power over my life—that I could control every element of every situation. I had never been able to work a compromise between those opposing sides, obviously because both were incomplete.

My life had been a game of asking others to take control, then becoming angry at the terrible job they did. In reaction, I would try to manage every little detail on my own, becoming even more furious to find that I had no more success than anyone else. That morning, as my desire to find a better way came screaming forth, I knew that I had to change my game or I would not survive.

Central to the power struggle was my ambivalence about God. I vacillated between "Yes, there is a God, and this is all His fault," and "There is no God, never has been, and never will be." The record running in my mind snagged on one thought: How could there be a God when my life and the lives of those around me were in such confusion?

It seemed clear to me that life was some kind of cruel joke, with people hanging around for the final punch line. Even though I was too fearful not to believe in God, I couldn't accept the idea that this life was just a trial period, a chance to earn a pass into heaven. Outrageous to think that all this suffering here on earth was just a prelude to finding joy with the angels above. I wanted no part of any heaven, any God, that allowed me to be so sick and miserable.

A favorite fantasy had me completing my time on earth, making it to Heaven's gates, and then being admitted by Saint Peter to join God. Each time, the fantasy ended with me saying "No, thanks" and walking away. But I really didn't have a lot of time to think about God. I was in too much pain.

Life as Battlefield

On my 27th birthday, no matter how terrified and confused I was, the reality I had fought for so long became very clear. I, Linda, was one of the living dead. Every morning I got up, went to work, came home, ate dinner, and went to bed; and each day was a replica of the days before it. The only joy in my life was my students, but after work I had to go home and be with myself. It isn't that wonderful things never happened in my life. It's just that I wouldn't have seen them if they had been standing on my nose.

Each day I drove home from work filled with feelings of emptiness, emptiness that began to fill me with intense anxiety. But instead of focusing on those feelings and what they were trying to tell me, I concentrated only on my physical pain. I couldn't face the fact that the problem was, and always had been, me. The pain was merely a result of the mental race I was losing.

So I got up each morning and did the same things over and over again. Over and over. Over and over. I had a pulse, but I was dead. The only thing that let me know I was still breathing was the chronic pain. It was the only sign of life my body gave me, the only part of my life that I allowed myself to feel.

What was this horrible life I had? By most standards, I had it all. I was well-educated, had a good job, handsome husband, caring family, home, friends—but none of this seemed to ease my pain. I added to my possessions, enrolled in a Ph.D. program, joined a spa—I grasped at anything external to solve a problem I couldn't even label.

About two months before the morning I woke up screaming, I began having panic attacks, moments of horror that struck quickly and seemed to last an eternity. Trying to force them to stop only made the problem worse. Because of the attacks, sitting through meetings at work became impossible, and dashing away from the dinner table was routine. I would find myself sitting in the bathroom gasping for air or throwing up whatever I had managed to eat. Driving became hazardous. I often pulled over to the side of the road to avoid deliberately driving into a telephone pole or running over a passing jogger who obviously knew nothing about pain.

I kept asking myself what was wrong—why was I acting this way? How dare I complain or feel anxious when so many of my friends were envious of what I had? Of what they thought I had. And, as I was frequently reminded, compared with other RA patients, I was doing okay.

About two months before my birthday and soon after the panic attacks began, I had asked my doctor to recommend a counselor. He insisted that I didn't need one. It was obvious to everyone how well I was coping with this disease. Why, I was working full time, managing a home, exercising, walking—doing much better than most of his other patients.

This was something I often confronted during my search for healing. Because other RA victims were perceived as sicker than I, it seemed that I had no right to want less pain, better medication, or the ability to run marathons. And because I was afraid to speak up for myself, other people ran my life. I allowed others to tell me what was appropriate and inappropriate for my body, and then walked around enraged because I had given away my power.

I tortured myself with questions like, "Don't they want me to get better?" "Don't I have the right to try to improve my health?" Now I realize that the people I was working with only reflected my own beliefs—it was I who didn't think I had a right to heal. I felt I was being punished (for what I wasn't sure) and that I was unworthy of health. Like my doctor, I was also a comparer. But while I measured myself against people who were healthy, my physician compared me only with invalids.

A Cry for Help

The day came when I could no longer contain my frustration at being denied emotional help. As my doctor and I went through our monthly debate about counseling, I burst into tears. They weren't much, but they were the best I could do. Weeping made me feel ugly, unlovable, and out of control but I couldn't help myself. At least, they did the trick.

My doctor, for all that he had seen me through—the pain, the slow, relentless erosion of my body—had never seen me cry. Although I was slowly losing the capacity to move, I had not allowed myself the comfort of crying in front of the person who was the primary caretaker of my illness. He was so impressed that I had an appointment with a psychiatrist within an hour.

A year later, I realized that I hadn't needed my doctor's permission to see a counselor. All it would have taken was a copy of the yellow pages and a few phone calls. Long afterwards, I was able to admit that I didn't want to take care of myself. I wanted him to do it for me.

Although the appointment with the psychiatrist was several weeks away, I felt calm for the first time in months. I needed the assurance that help was on its way, because life as I knew it was falling apart and I knew I couldn't get through it alone. In 27 years, I had been unable to change. Not being too sure about God, I saw a psychiatrist as my only other option.

Who Is This Person?

By now, my home life was also a disaster. I had always been the rock in our marriage, stoic and totally responsible. Seeing me so distraught made my husband happy to know I was human on the one hand, and scared to death on the other.

As the focus of our relationship changed and I began to confront my life, it struck me that we had spent all our time worrying about his problems. My needs had rarely been a topic of discussion between us, although we both knew I was becoming more physically disabled each day. As I began to struggle with the task of unraveling who I had become, the only support my husband could give me was to rehearse the bleak history of mental illness in my family. His reminder brought out fears of nervous breakdown and ongoing mental illness that had followed me since childhood.

We tried to communicate, but our most trivial differences remained unresolved, and we realized that we would have to work hard to change. During this time, we also confronted the fact that we had little in common except our unhappiness and our inability to support each other. After a few half-hearted attempts to resolve some of our issues, we stopped trying. Without the commitment to interact lovingly, even the meager amount of communication that had existed between us began to fade, along with any desire to stay together and work things out.

And Who Are All These Others?

My life with my parents and sisters was also unraveling. I had always visited my parents once or twice a week. My intention was to change them, to get them to see and do things my way. I was a pain in the neck, but at least I made my presence known. When I finally admitted that I had problems in my own life, I lost interest in theirs. In a matter of moments, my attention was gone.

My sisters and I had always loved and cared for each other, but in many ways our relationships were equally shallow. Here again, although I was dependent on their love, I knew something had to change. I began to withdraw from them angrily. My brother and I had never been close. With him, I did what I had always done: I tried my best to ignore him.

At the same time, I was also beginning to admit problems with my career. Much time and money had been spent training me to do a job that did not fulfill my creative needs. And equally important, how could I continue to work in a helping field when I was unable to help myself? I knew it often happened this way and saw it all around me—people "helping" other people when they couldn't stand themselves. But knowing this did not ease my new-found desire to change. The small part of me that wanted a different life was beginning to demand attention.

The question, "How do people change?" reverberated through my skull. I couldn't understand how change was possible. My life had been consistently miserable, but at least that misery had a certain stability. As things stood now, I had no idea what was coming next. Knowing that I had an appointment with a psychiatrist gave me the strength to get through the next few weeks. It was a great relief to know that someone was going to help, even though I wasn't at all sure what that meant.

III. DECIDING TO CHANGE

For the sake of clarity, I would like to describe the disease that seemed to cause all my problems. My description is different from the ones you read in medical books. Those definitions don't describe people who have rheumatoid arthritis (RA), they describe the medical symptoms. I'll try to do a little of both.

• **Rheumatoid Arthritis.** Disease. Believed to be stress related.

• **"No known cure,"** therefore, a disease of hopelessness.

• **Chronic pain.** Like being taken by the hair and slammed against a brick wall. Nonstop. No matter what anyone says, you never get used to pain.

• **Hands, feet, knees don't work.** It's a struggle to get from point A to point B hoping people won't ask what's wrong, knowing that they will.

• **Swelling and disfigurement.** Hiding your hands so no one grabs them and says, "Gosh, what happened to you?"

• **Fatigue.** Longing for the hour when you can just get into bed and sleep. (Bedtime comes earlier each night.)

• **Sleep.** If the pain will let you. Be sure to take enough pills.

• **Depression.** Hopelessness, lack of self worth. Why go on?

• **Loneliness.** No one understands. Why go on?

• **Helplessness.** There's no way to get better. Why go on?

• **Dry eyes and mouth**. There's no water in my eyes. Can't blink without drops every five minutes. Fake saliva—spray it in so I can swallow.

• **Medications.** So, doctor, what are "we" trying this week?

•**Addiction to pain killers.** Just give me something—anything— to knock me out.

• **Loss of appetite.** All I want to do is sleep. Who cares about food?

• **Etc.**

So Where Was I?

The psychiatrist's office was disappointing; I had imagined it in a different building. (Once again, I managed to shield myself in trivia by worrying about the building.) I took a test; he asked me questions; I lied. I stuck to my old story—everything in my life was great except this disease. It had brought me there, and if it would just go away, my life would be complete.

This went on for months. I didn't tell him about any problems except those related to RA, but knowing that someone was concerned about me gave me strength to move quickly in other areas. And something about the therapy situation itself gave me reassurance. I showed up every week and not only was he there, the furniture was always in place and he didn't fall asleep when I decided to talk. This very supportive man encouraged me just by his presence.

Moving Out, Moving On

Two months after I started therapy, I decided that my husband and I had to work on our marriage or I was leaving. One month later I moved out, and it was a relief. Our marriage was like my job: I had been trained to be married, but being trained and being happy were two different issues.

I had always craved crisis situations, but the constant chaos of our marriage had left me exhausted. Our breakup gave me more time and energy to deal with my illness. During the next therapy session after I moved out, my psychiatrist noted that I hadn't even told him I was having marital problems until I was ready to pack my bags.

So three months after I had looked at myself in the mirror and seen myself as if for the first time, I had started therapy and my marriage was over. Well, I thought, things were finally going to get better.

I was wrong. After all the pain I had already been through, I had no idea of the pain to come. If anyone had told me about the agony of the next three years, I would have laughed and called him a liar. It was time for me to heal. I was convinced I was on my way up—the pain would leave, probably within the next 30 minutes. After 27 years of negative thinking and living a life of self-condemnation, I should have known that healing would take a little time.

I was embarking on a project that I now call "re-learning to think." During this time, I realized how ignorant I was when it came to healing. My embarrassment left me so tired that at times, I didn't want to go on. Now when I begin to condemn myself, I remind myself that the pain is gone and I'm still here, but then it wasn't as easy.

After I moved out of the house I shared with my husband, I rented a room instead of finding my own place. I really wasn't sure what I wanted to do or where I wanted to go and in truth, I wasn't ready to be alone. I didn't want a companion or any real communication, I just wanted to know that someone was near. Old habits die hard.

For all the work I had to do, I was moving very quickly. But all I remember is how slowly the days seemed to pass. I started timing myself when I got dressed because I was sure three hours had lapsed between putting on my socks and tying my shoes. When I prepared my meals, I kept asking myself how long a frozen dinner could take. I was aware of myself and the moment I was in for the first time, and I didn't like it. Living in the past or the future were the only things I knew how to do.

I kept asking myself if what I had was better than what I had left. The difficulty I had answering this question truly annoyed me. In fact, I wasn't sure what I had left. Living in reality had never been my strong point. I did what I had to do, then retreated into a shell of fantasy. I didn't really know what my husband was like. I wasn't sure who I was. Twenty seven years—wasted.

Now, by any sensible account, I had accomplished a lot in those 27 years. But I had removed myself from my life—in my mind, I hadn't done anything. It had all just happened. It felt like a lie to say that I had participated in any of this activity. The only feelings I remembered with any clarity about the first 27 years of my life were confusion and physical pain. So here I was at age 27 still filled with pain, but much less confused. Without the confusion, I was now free to live in the moment, but I had no idea what to do.

The Pact

I didn't like my new home, but I really had nothing to compare it with. I had never felt comfortable anywhere. I was still in a job that didn't fit. My family and I were not doing well. And I was getting sicker by the minute. But during this time of slow motion, I made the decision that would change my life forever. I made a written agreement to give myself five years. I would either get well, or I would kill myself.

Calmly, I wrote out this agreement, signed it, put it in an envelope, and went to sleep. I told no one about it, not even my psychiatrist. It was the only thing I had ever done that was my own. It was the only time I had ever been instrumental in a decision that would have a major effect on my life. I couldn't blame anyone for this except me. But who puts herself on a five-year death plan when a six-month schedule would have saved a lot of time? Why didn't I just get the whole thing over with quickly?

It is clear to me now that I wanted to live, but I couldn't have been convinced of that at the time I made the pact. It was my sincere intention to see the plan through to the end—no matter what the outcome. Although I was willing to try everything I could, I remained convinced that nothing would work. The hopeless, helpless side of me was still running the show.

But somewhere inside me was another person who thought maybe I could do it. Without realizing it, I had taken my first steps toward healing long before writing the pact. My desire to live and live joyfully was much stronger than I had ever consciously imagined.

The next morning, I looked at the envelope and reaffirmed my commitment to try. Then I did something that I had been wanting to do for a long time. I drove to a nearby cemetery and walked slowly and intently to a grave that couldn't be seen from the road. I laid on top of the grave and tried to imagine what it was like to be dead. A satisfying feeling crept through me as I realized that after I was buried, my bones would return to dust. Maybe they would do more good for the soil of the earth than they had ever done for me.

Besides, bones made of dust couldn't hurt.

IV. MAKING A LIST

My activities during the weeks to come were typical—just the type of behavior that I desperately wanted to change. As I struggled with ways to attack the demon disease that was attacking me, I limited myself to two "tried and failed" approaches: 1) get other people to do what had to be done or 2) do it all myself. In my mind, there were no shades of grey—only black and white. My psychiatrist called this "All or nothing thinking." I now call it "A great way to waste time."

Words on Paper

I was confused and unable to make decisions. I knew that what I was doing wasn't working, although I didn't know why. I also knew my frustration level was reaching its peak and I needed to do something quickly. A million ideas whirled in my mind but I couldn't focus on any of them. In my uncertainty and confusion, I finally decided that I needed to make a list.

Writing down what I wanted to try was a good way to validate the ideas spinning in my head. Although that piece of paper represented only random thoughts, I valued it. It was tangible evidence that there were things I could do.

After I allowed myself a certain amount of time to feel relieved about making the list, I panicked again. Now that I had it, how was I going to deal with it? In the end, I decided to set up some guidelines or rules to help me cope. There were only four, but they made me feel better about the list:

1. The only way I could modify the list would be to add to it.

2. I did not have to start at the beginning of the list and work down. I could do whatever I wanted to do in any order.

3. There were no time limits for starting or completing any item, but I did need to keep my five-year deadline in mind.

4. If I tried something on the list and doing it really annoyed me, I could put it aside and go on to something else. But eventually, I had to try each item.

When I made those rules, it didn't occur to me that I was taking an amazing step in the right direction. I made the rules; I would follow them. In doing so, I had also given up some of the negative control I had always placed on myself. I was saying that I wouldn't give up, a least for a certain period of time.

I was relieved and a little proud that the list started with something I had already begun: therapy. I did remind myself that I had only gone into therapy because I felt that I was losing control, not because I wanted to improve my life.

Other people with RA seemed more accepting of the lives they shared with the disease—they didn't seem to get emotionally upset or lose control as I did. Their conversations focused on two major concepts: first, "Ain't it awful?" and second, "We're stuck with this, so let's do what the doctor says."

My tendency was to join the crowd who felt they weren't well because someone had messed up their treatment. (It was difficult to find people who would openly blame their current doctors, but earlier doctors took a lot of heat.) The trouble with blaming was that it made me feel better for only a few minutes, then I was back where I started. Although I couldn't force myself to accept the hand that life had dealt me, I began to realize that if I were satisfied with suffering silently or complaining in a reasonable manner, I wouldn't have started therapy or made the pact.

At one point, the breakup of my marriage seemed like something I could add to the list as a success. But somewhere inside, I wasn't sure that a divorce was anything to work for or be proud of, so I left it off. By now I was tuned in enough to know that simply leaving my husband had not solved the problems we shared. Another sobering fact about the separation was that the pain and disease had not vanished when I left. Indeed, both were getting worse.

And what were the items on my list? Here goes:

- individual therapy
- group therapy
- Alexander Technique
- meditation
- AA
- swimming or water exercise
- physical therapy
- occupational therapy
- a writing course
- a new career
- acupuncture
- biofeedback
- self-help books

- diet
- affirmations
- vitamin therapy
- voice lessons
- dream work
- autogenics
- visualization
- releasing myself from people who were bullies
- deciding what I thought about God

At that point, I couldn't imagine leaving the realm of traditional medicine. The doctor stayed on my mental list as a necessity.

There were a few more items on the original list; I can't remember all of them now. I do recall spending about five minutes writing the list, then sitting back and being surprised at how easy it was. I couldn't remember ever consciously considering any of these methods except individual counseling, group therapy, and biofeedback, the first because I was already involved and the second and third because my psychiatrist had recommended them.

I had been assembling the list in my mind for a long time.

Ticking off the Items

Finally I began to deal with my list and my pact. The pattern was simple—first a cycle of frantic activity, then a pause for rest and panic. At least it was a new approach to solving my problems. I had never worked through anything before; it was easier to give up before I started. Soon, however, I managed to reach an activity level that left no time for the rest/panic part of the cycle. I kept moving for the next four years, and then slept 12 to 15 hours a day for three months.

I had already started one of the activities on my list. My insurance covered individual therapy, once a week. Group therapy was out of the question because it wasn't covered. My next choices were to begin reading self-help books and taking a writing class. My employers would pay for the class, as I did a lot of writing in my job. Taking the course gave me immense pleasure but I was constantly concerned that I would fail or be asked to withdraw. These failure fantasies opened another Pandora's box: I had always refused to try anything that really interested me because I knew that I would fail. Instead, I only did things I felt fairly secure about—which wasn't a lot.

Because of my work in the writing class, other activities I had wanted to try began to crowd my mind—longings that had never before seen the light of day. I had to face my conviction that if I couldn't do something perfectly the first time, I would never succeed. In my mind, creative people didn't have to work at what they did. Their creations came as easily as snapping their fingers. Still, even with all these feelings of unworthiness, I pressed on.

I picked up a magazine article on affirmations and decided to try writing them. The affirmations did not seem to challenge my irresponsibility directly, but soon I realized that they did. My life wasn't even close to the affirmations I was using, and it was unclear to me how to reach the goals. I did the recommended exercises for a while, probably a week or two. My mistrust of the future and the fact that I didn't see dramatic results immediately gave me reason to stop.

Of course, it may have been that the examples in the article were designed for people who were pretty sophisticated in the affirmation game, which I was not. All they did for me was enhance my hopelessness and anxiety. I dropped affirmations to the bottom of the list, but four years later I began using them again. Saying, "I approve of myself," was much easier than saying, "I am now perfect in all ways." Approving of myself wasn't as easy as I thought, but four years later, I was ready to try.

Each day I became more involved in the details of the pact. When complications arose, I treated them as evils. I kept telling myself that it was okay; this was only for a certain period of time, then I could call it quits. And yet another part of me was beginning to enjoy the game.

Money Matters

After I made the rules for dealing with my list, it dawned on me that I had to find a way to support the plan financially. It seemed that if I didn't worry about where to get the money, my dream of healing would never become a reality. I knew that I had to make a firm financial commitment to healing, beyond just deciding that it was going to cost me an incredible amount of money. Each time I read over the list, the money issue loomed to the surface. After much inner debate, I finally made an agreement that every cent I earned for the next five years would have to support my goal of getting well. I didn't like that part of the deal, but I made it anyway.

Spending the next five years paying a debt I never felt I owed didn't appeal to me. Money was something I hadn't worried a lot about until I decided to get well. Before that time, it was just one more concept stashed away in the back of my mind. Confronting and taking care of my own financial needs would have meant taking responsibility for myself, a responsibility I still believed belonged to my parents. (I would never have admitted that at the time but it was true.) Even when I was married and working full-time, I always thought of them as my financial backup if something should happen.

Financial dependence might have been an upsetting thought, but I was much more comfortable with the word "dependence" than the word "freedom." As I confronted an issue I had managed to avoid all my adult life, I was no longer merely upset but enraged. How had I lived on the earth for 28 years without developing the ability to take care of myself? I was determined to work this problem through and replace dependence with freedom.

As I estimated how much it would cost to get well, I began to assume that it would be hard for me to get the money and that whatever I got would not be enough. I saw clearly that there was a difference between what I wanted and what I was getting. I sensed that the freedom I longed for was out of reach unless I learned to do many things differently.

In the meantime, the list of professionals willing to help me in my quest for healing got longer, as did the bills they sent me each month. My growing awareness led me to realize that I always paid some of those bills in full (sometimes in advance). There were others that I had been paying for years, and would still be paying years later. I understood that I was willing to pay in full for what I believed was helping me, but not for what I wasn't sure was worth my time or money. Soon after, it dawned on me that this principle applied to all my financial transactions, not just those involving my body.

During this time I also realized that there was no way a person in my frame of mind could attract what she thought she wanted. If I had been able to develop the kind of mind that easily attracted abundance, I probably wouldn't have been sick in the first place. And I finally acknowledged that I must have been angry about financial issues for years. It had always been a major problem between my husband and myself, although we never discussed it openly until the end of our marriage. I saw that it was time for me to give money and the role it played in my life the attention it deserved.

The money dilemma brought up yet another familiar behavior pattern that tied in with my feelings of unworthiness: comparing myself with other people. What was wrong with me that I couldn't easily raise the money I needed? Other people seemed to get money without blinking an eye. Fortunately, even as I wallowed around in anger, I was able to decide what I wanted to try next. I woke up each day with mixed feelings of hopelessness and excitement as I planned my next move.

The Alexander Technique

A friend at work had been going to weekly sessions to learn the Alexander Technique. After talking with her about it, I decided that my next financial investment toward becoming healthy would be weekly sessions with a certified instructor, an item that was not covered by insurance. The monetary aspect annoyed me, but since I hadn't tried the technique, I didn't let myself move it to the end of the list. I found that each time I chose an item that cost more than a dollar, it brought up my money issues. I would struggle with them again and again.

I mentioned trying the Alexander Technique to my physician and I was surprised when he gave me his complete support. He had known other patients who had benefitted greatly from learning and working with the technique. His reaction encouraged me even more, and I started going once a week.

Two books about the Alexander Technique are listed in the resource section. I recommend reading them or taking an introductory seminar to learn about the method. The simplest way I can describe the technique is "ease of posture and movement." I learned new ways to move my body that put the smallest amount of stress on my joints and muscles. Instead of constantly contorting my body to avoid pain, I learned to lengthen my limbs in the direction of my movements.

My Alexander teacher kept assuring me that I caught on to the principles very quickly—I was one of her best students. It seemed hard for her to grasp the intensity of my pain. It made me feel much better to use my body in the ways she taught me. I practiced going up and down stairs, opening and closing doors, sitting down and getting up from the toilet and various kinds of chairs, lying down, walking across the room, turning faucets on and off, standing still, putting on clothes and taking them off, leaning over to pick things up—everything. And every movement was a new kind of pain.

To explain why this technique helped so much, it is necessary to understand how I reacted to the pain in my body. If my left foot hurt, I would put all my weight on the right side of my body, a natural reaction. When a healthy person does this, it's not good but it's not disastrous, either. Sooner or later the left foot stops hurting and things get back to normal.

With RA, things don't get back to normal, and walking around like that only makes the right foot start hurting. The pain is cyclical and unending. It moves from the right foot to the left and back again. Most of the time, both feet hurt at the same time. What occurs is a constant contortion of the body to cushion the pain of almost any movement. When I realized that the way I moved added to the pain in my body, I became very motivated to change.

The Alexander Technique is the kind of treatment that brings immediate and positive effects for people who are well motivated and involved with a competent instructor. I was both. Because of these quick, positive results, it was one of my best choices from the list. I continued to integrate Alexander Techniques into my life until I became so sick that every breath I took was a nightmare. When the pain reached a certain magnitude, I lost interest in moving at all.

I was now spending two evenings a week and one Saturday a month dealing with RA on the physical level, and every spare moment thinking about it. It was the beginning of a physical and mental purge that would take me on what seemed like a descent straight into hell.

I began to feel that the process of change had split me open and that I was seeping out, oozing out all over the place. I felt myself slipping and sliding in my own insides as I tried to walk, but was still unable to accept that this oozing mess was my responsibility. It was still impossible for me to understand that my physical illness had been created by the way I unconsciously chose to think day after day, year after year. I was exhausted, infuriated, confused, and in more pain with each passing minute, but I was determined to see this pact through to the end.

V. RA AND ME

Rheumatoid arthritis first found me in 1974. I woke up one morning with a stiff, red, swollen finger on my right hand. Nothing like that had ever happened to my hands before, although my right ankle had been in a cast the year before. Again, that had been a matter of waking up one morning with a swollen, stiff ankle that would not heal. When friends asked what had happened I lied, saying that I had tripped and sprained it. Actually, nothing had happened. My ankle simply wouldn't work. After the cast was removed, the pain went away and I didn't give it another thought.

The pain in my finger also went away after a few days and I resumed life as normal. Two weeks later, I woke up with the same problem in the corresponding finger of my left hand. Again, it went away and I quit thinking about it. Two weeks later, I woke up unable to use any of the fingers in either hand. That day I finally realized that I had a problem. I went to the college infirmary, they took a blood test, and it came back positive for RA.

The college physician sent me to specialists. After two days of testing, the doctors reported that although the tests were inconclusive, they believed I had lupus. Back in 1974, lupus was considered a killer. Back on campus with what I felt was a death sentence hanging over my head, I continued with my studies. I neither asked for nor received any counseling, nor did I follow up on any medical care.

Nothing much happened for a while except that I walked around becoming more and more depressed. Considering that I was already refusing to deal with a life-long depression, things weren't going very well at all. I wandered through the days doing my school work, one day feeling enraged, the next hopeless.

Over Thanksgiving break that year, I went to a baby shower. Talking with the woman sitting next to me, I found out that she worked for a rheumatologist, or a doctor who specialized in arthritis. She had noticed immediately that I didn't look well and asked what the problem was. I told her what I knew, which wasn't much. She was horrified to find that I was not on medication and had not been to a doctor since my quasi-diagnosis. She almost insisted that I make an appointment with one of the doctors in the practice where she worked.

My Doctor, My Friend

I had my first appointment with the doctor one month later. After another series of blood tests, he reported that there was no question in his mind. I did not have lupus; I had rheumatoid arthritis. I had walked around for a year and a half thinking I was dead meat for nothing.

His recommendation was to begin a rigorous series of gold treatments and aspirin immediately. I started receiving gold injections, and I quickly worked up to 27 aspirins a day. I wasn't sure how well the gold was working, but the aspirin made me feel great. I had been concerned about taking aspirin because of my earlier stomach ulcer, but they didn't bother me at all. I felt better than I had in two years. Back at college, I found a doctor who was willing to give me a gold shot once a week. I proceeded to get gold injections and down 27 aspirins or more every day for the next six years.

During those next six years, a lot happened in my life. I earned my bachelor's and master's degrees, got married, bought a house, and pretended to carry on with life. I vaguely remember being physically present for those events—even signing up for them—but I was not emotionally involved in any aspect of my life except to express anger and hopelessness. Those years were foggy, hazy. I got up reluctantly, day after day, and did what I had to do. Like a reed, I blew in whatever direction the wind took me; did whatever was most socially acceptable. Not that I was easy to get along with; I was always looking for and finding situations that gave me a chance to be angry.

What's Wrong With Me?

Although I usually felt okay, I began having trouble with my eyes. They were dry and scratchy, to the extent that I couldn't wear my contact lenses comfortably. It finally became painful for me to wear lenses for more than four hours at a time. The insides of my eyelids began to feel like double-sided sandpaper, and each time I blinked the sandpaper would rub against the lids and eyeballs.

I was used to wearing contact lenses from sunup to sundown, so I knew something was seriously wrong. Finally, an ophthalmologist told me that if I continued I would risk rupturing my corneas and losing my vision, so I threw out the contacts. I found out that I had Sjogren's Syndrome, a condition directly related to RA, that dries out the natural fluids of both the eyes and mouth. My mouth had not been affected yet, but I was terrified that a disease I thought only affected my joints could also destroy my vision and my ability to enjoy the taste of food.

Time went on, and then the bottom fell out. I had an especially stressful day teaching (most of them were) and was gearing up for a long afternoon when my aide pointed out that my face had become red and blotchy. I realized that along with a hot, swollen face, I was having trouble breathing. It is still hard for me to accept that although strange things kept happening in my body, I only reacted to them when someone else noticed.

I raced out of the classroom and called my doctor, who told me to get to the nearest emergency room. I was having an allergic reaction to aspirin. By the time I reached the hospital, I was tearing my clothes off in panic, unable to breathe. My doctor had called ahead and as I ran into the emergency room, someone grabbed me and injected adrenaline. Then benedryl. Then more adrenaline. Then more benedryl. As my allergist explained later, I had reacted to aspirin in the same way that some people react to bee stings. He taught me how to give myself a shot if I had to, because he was afraid that it might happen again. Not wanting to argue the point, I began carrying a syringe of adrenaline in my purse at all times.

No More Aspirin?

The upshot of that particular drama was that I could not consider ever putting another aspirin down my throat. When I asked the allergist about it, he looked at me as if I was crazy. He said he hadn't given me the syringe to carry around in my purse for nothing—that another aspirin would probably lead to the same reaction. If I did decide to take aspirin again, he said I should do myself a favor and take it near an emergency room.

As I drove home, my head filled with visions of screaming, I didn't allow myself the release of doing so in reality. How could he tell me such a thing? Didn't he understand that I needed aspirin to exist? How would I get through the pain? What would keep the swelling down? I was sure that now the disease would surge untamed through my body and I would become a cripple. I was still getting gold injections, but by now was questioning their value. How could I live without aspirin?

I remember consciously separating myself from my body, even from the turmoil in my mind—simply vacating the premises of my own existence. When I got home my husband asked how the appointment had gone. As if I had just been to the drug store to pick up some toothpaste, I replied that everything was fine; I just couldn't take aspirin any more. That was the end of the discussion.

Without the incredible amounts of aspirin I had been taking, and probably because I believed it would, the arthritis flourished. In desperation, I tried anti-cancer and anti-malarial drugs, medications better known for their side effects than for their healing abilities. My body would not tolerate them.

The Golden Cage

By that time I was getting gold injections on a monthly basis. Gold is a toxic substance that the body can not eliminate, and my doctor watched me closely for signs of toxicity. Of course I had them. Not only did I experience rashes and sores in my mouth, I also itched constantly, all over my body.

Because of those reactions, he began spacing the gold shots further and further apart. Even without obvious symptoms, decreasing the frequency of shots is the accepted pattern in gold therapy. When my body began to reject the other medications, I asked him to start increasing the frequency of gold injections again. The reactions and the RA just got worse, but I continued to have the shots as often as I could. I was afraid not to. What else was there?

By that time, I was in a constant state of fury. My entire existence revolved around my deteriorating physical health. All the attention I received from my family and friends centered on whatever was the latest disaster with RA. After 20 years of being sick, it was all I knew how to do. The web surrounding me became thicker and more dense until even the possibility for health of body and mind was lost in the work of spiders who were weaving me into madness.

I began to wonder if I would reach my 30th birthday. Did I want to reach my 30th birthday? Was there any point in my continued existence? Why go on?

VI. ONE STEP FORWARD, THREE STEPS BACK

About a year before my husband and I separated, I did something that was a perfect example of the way I chose to ignore my physical needs. I took a job working with deaf students in an institution that required constant use of sign language. In this job, my hands would be busy with intricate, fine motor movements eight hours a day. The program was residential, and it was assumed that I would help with after-school activities as well as teach a full load. To do both would mean abusing my hands for at least 10 hours a day.

Now I understand that even applying for the job was an act of self-destruction. I was becoming more physically disabled by the moment, and I had deliberately placed the most severely affected parts of my body in a situation where they would literally fall apart.

My attempts to change my life in this manner continued until I understood that I couldn't solve my inner problems by altering outward circumstances. I constantly bought new things, thinking that each one would make some important difference. I expected each new dress or new kind of makeup to ease the part of me that was hurting, but it never happened. Because I felt worthless, anything I owned for more than an hour became worthless, too.

Long afterward, I began to understand that I didn't need to change my style of dress, I needed to change my style of thinking; I didn't need to change the way I looked, but the way I felt; I didn't need to change my job, only my attitudes about work. Finally, I didn't need to take on a second job to earn more money, I needed to confront and change the feelings about money that were keeping me at the edge of bankruptcy. But that day was still far off in the future. Until then, nothing I possessed made "the difference." And my exciting new job was like a new dress—once I had it, I didn't want it. I had moments of joy and success with my students, but they were not enough to ease the pain.

After I accepted the job and discovered that I was still unhappy, I knew that seeking yet another job was not the answer. I stayed and functioned as well as I could, refusing to become involved with anything but the two most essential activities: teaching and going to meetings. My peers were very much involved in their students' lives and I felt guilty for not doing more.

My inability to make the connection between mind and body, along with the constant strain on my hands, left me no time to tackle any more items on the list. I had other things to worry about. The joint in the index finger of my right hand was the first fatality of the war raging inside me.

Falling Apart

It became almost impossible to use my index finger and when I did, the pain was incredible. At one routine visit, I told my doctor that I was in severe pain and was forcing myself to use my hands at work. On the drive home, I could barely hold on to the steering wheel. The pain and swelling even made it difficult for me to care for myself.

After the aspirin experience, I had tried just about every other medication my doctor could name. There were no more treatments available to me except pain killers—nothing would stop or slow the progression of the disease. For lack of other options, he reluctantly recommended joint replacement.

I made an appointment with a surgeon and as I walked into his office, I knew that I was now considered "very sick." Joint replacement was the last resort for people with this disease, and here I was, about to sign up. Looking around the waiting room, I saw people like myself but I refused to place myself among them. In my need to be separate, I had become very skilled at noticing differences instead of similarities.

The surgeon could tell without an X-ray that the joint was gone. He recommended replacement surgery as soon as possible. I wanted to see the X-ray and think about it some more. But as soon as I saw the X-ray, I knew there really wasn't much of a decision to make. All that was left of the joint was a thin sliver of mushy cartilage surrounded by disease. Now I knew why I hadn't been able to use the finger. There was no joint left to use. I set the date without getting a second opinion.

It seemed very clear that this disease would continue to rampage through my body no matter what drug I swallowed or had injected. People frequently remarked that I was too young to be so sick, but I felt very old. I had lost interest in my list, even in practicing the Alexander Technique. The breakdown of my marriage, and the issues surrounding it took the back burner, although I did continue with therapy. All I thought about was the part of my body that I was trading in for a piece of plastic.

Water had always been a soothing element in my life. The morning before my surgery, in dire need of comfort, I attempted to wash some of my troubles away by going to the swimming pool. I lowered myself into the water, pleased that I had finally found my way to a bit of peace. I did two strokes through the water, then stopped when I heard something snap. I stood up in the water and looked around to see what part of me had floated off. Knowing that the sound had come from the right side of my body, I reached into the water and pulled out the useless appendage that had once been my right hand and wrist.

There is a bone (unnecessary for everything but cosmetic purposes) between the wrist and the hand. At some point—I had no idea when—that bone had literally split in half. The main tendon running through my hand, wrist, and arm had become lodged in the split, and had gradually been severed because of the constant wear and tear of movement through the broken bone. Those few strokes in the pool had given it the final push. I don't remember any pain at the time it snapped but when I realized what had happened, I almost drowned myself.

Using my left hand, I managed to get out of the pool, dress myself, and drive home. As I drove, I was haunted once again by the belief that I was unfit to live, and that I didn't want to. The next day, the surgeon told me how fortunate it was that this had happened all at once. Lucky me; I wouldn't have to come back in a month for more surgery. I was not impressed.

Before and After

The results of the operation were minimal. Scar tissue formed quickly around the incision, freezing the tendons. I had no follow-up physical or occupational therapy. Despite surgery, the joint was still not usable.

When the swelling went down, I finally got a good look at my hand and wrist. The "before-after" pictures on the surgeon's wall had not prepared me for what I saw. Before me was an appendage that belonged to a creature from another planet. Two additional joints in my pinky had frozen in the cast, leaving other previously uninvolved joints useless as well. I remember saying "this is not my hand, this is not my hand" over and over, hoping that by denying its presence, it would disappear.

The one positive outcome was no more pain in my finger and wrist. This was a big relief. I still had use of the middle and ring fingers and the thumb of that hand, but even so, I was furious about the results of the surgery. I kept my rage to myself, once again putting off dealing with my most urgent feelings. The rage continued to grow inside me, literally paralyzing my body.

After surgery I faced the ordeal of caring for myself with my left, non-dominant hand. It took everything I had just to survive. Although I had been in pain before, taking care of myself had never been a problem except when I had an arthritis attack. During the two days of a typical attack, I needed someone to care for me. Then I would be all right again for months at a time. The attacks rarely threatened my feelings of independence because they were short and infrequent. I compared an attack to a cold or the flu, and took my ability to care for myself for granted. Until I was unable to take aspirin and had surgery, I didn't believe that I could become a cripple. It might happen to other people, but not to me. I had considered suicide because I didn't want to live with illness, not because I couldn't hold a toothbrush long enough to brush my teeth.

But this recuperation period was different. All of the independence I had taken for granted seemed like a dream from another life. My reality was a nightmare. The surgery had placed me in a situation where I was forced to ask for help. Even the simplest activity took twice as long to accomplish. I was unable to feed, clothe, or bathe myself without assistance. If I wanted to go for a walk, I had to wait for someone to come home and tie my shoes. If I wanted to go anywhere, I had to arrange for someone to drive me. As the days wore on, my feelings of anger and worthlessness mounted. Most people having any kind of surgery expect to be helpless for a while. Not me. The reality of my situation did not hit me until I was in the middle of it.

Things at work had also become complex. I had resumed teaching a week after surgery, with my right hand and arm in a cast. I had no option but to sign with my left hand. This was not easy but I managed. My students, my colleagues, and the administrators of the program were very supportive and I carried on as if nothing had happened.

I recovered, slowly, but now there was a new problem. My left hand, now doing the work of both hands, began to feel as bad as the right one did before the surgery.

I had always exhibited an air of bravado and independence, but behind this aura was really a frightened child. The experience of having to depend on other people pushed my opposing needs for independence and support to the surface. A physical sensation of spinning in the eye of a tornado tormented me—awake or dreaming. The tornado seemed to be carrying me to a place and time where I could understand that I did need other people to survive—not only during illness, but during times of health.

A Place to Live

Finally I was well enough to stop depending on others for my daily existence. No longer confronted with the logistics of survival, I found myself dealing with an issue that these months of being incapacitated had brought to the surface. Staying in someone else's home intensified my fears. "Dependency" was a dirty word. I didn't believe anyone else could take care of me, and I had already proved that I couldn't do it myself.

To compound the situation, I had filed for divorce. My temporary living arrangements no longer made any sense. As I came closer to being able to care for myself again, I realized that I did not want to go back to where I had lived before the surgery. The possibility of reconciling with my husband had kept me from getting my own place, but by now it was clear that the marriage was over. It was long past time for me to decide where I wanted to live.

I wanted to live on my own but didn't think I could. First, the thought of being alone terrified me. Secondly, I believed I couldn't afford it. For these two reasons, I decided to rent an apartment with a friend. It turned out to be a less than perfect arrangement, but I was happier there than I had been anywhere before. My roommate and I chose to share an apartment out of friendship, not desperation. We were both going through divorces, so we understood each other's problems. I shared more with her than I had with any friend or family member for a long time, including my husband. We even had fun together, quite a different experience for me. Making that move was a step in the right direction.

VII. ANOTHER YEAR ON THE BATTLEFIELD

Despite the many things that kept happening, the next year seemed like at least ten. Two people continued to live inside me, the one who had found the strength to write a list of options and the other who didn't go a week without considering suicide. They were still at war, but by now, the sides were at least equal in power.

Each day I faced that list—written by my own hand—that nagged at me to change my life. I must have read it a thousand times. The items that required the hardest inner work stayed on the bottom. Only the plans that involved getting someone else to teach me how to get better seemed possible. It may have been my 500th glance at the list when reality struck: no matter how much I paid for support, I had to do the real work myself. Therapy, of any kind, was not a life-long prescription. There had to come a day when I could take charge of my own health and my own life without paying anyone to help me. That time was still far off, but until it arrived, I had my pact, my list, and a growing desire to try.

On days when I felt a little stronger, I'd let myself glance toward the most disturbing item on the list: "A new career."

Had I really written that? I was well trained as a speech pathologist. I had a good job and was really quite successful. What else could I do? Who was I trying to kid? I wanted to write—but nobody got paid for doing what she wanted. Certainly not me. I desperately wanted to scratch that item off the list, but my rule was no erasing. Until I chose to address the issue of changing careers, it could stay at the bottom, but I could not remove it. Rules were rules.

Looking back, I understand why the thought of a new career made me panicky. In the three years after I earned my master's degree, I had worked in three different places. Each job left me more unhappy than the one before. I knew instinctively that it was destructive to spend 40 hours of every week doing something I didn't really want to do, but I felt trapped. I had watched several of my friends leave their full-time jobs to pursue creative dreams. In almost every case they did not succeed and had to return, at least temporarily, to their lackluster jobs. I watched some of them give up and never try again, and was sure the same thing would happen to me.

As painful as it was, I am now thankful that I had the opportunity to witness their experiences. It was one time that fear served as a positive motivator for me. Eventually I would be able to deal with my need for creative work, but only after I had developed some trust in myself.

Making another change before I was ready would have meant postponing success, and at that time, I would have interpreted delay as failure. So I continued to write, but the idea of writing as a career seemed a grossly impractical fantasy.

Exploring Terror

The events of the past two years combined with the unacknowledged inner work that I was doing began to leave me with "terror attacks" that were much worse than any panic attacks I had ever experienced. The old panic attacks had passed quickly; after I started therapy, they subsided completely. These new attacks stayed with me for long periods of time and left me exhausted. As their frequency increased, I stayed home whenever I could. Losing control in public did not appeal to me. I told no one about them because I was embarrassed.

Therapy was the only activity I had maintained consistently during the first few months after surgery, and by now I was being more open with my psychiatrist. Before I started therapy, there had been no way for me to show my feelings or even to admit that I had them. Even if I disliked someone intensely, or felt that I was being mistreated, I tried hard to keep peace by keeping silent.

I became adept at avoiding direct confrontations and tearing other people apart behind their backs. I changed opinions quickly and easily, depending on whom I was with at the time. Of course it's impossible to play both sides of every story, but I really believed that no one felt my deceit. It was obvious to everyone but me.

Admitting to and sharing my feelings felt dangerous. The most threatening thing to me was the fear of being abandoned, and I knew that the only way I could take care of myself was by keeping everyone else happy. To me, the problem was simple: I must never express my feelings honestly, or I would be left alone.

Until therapy, it hadn't occurred to me that I could develop into the kind of person who could create positive situations and attract people who could honestly handle emotions. I learned that there were ways to take care of myself without losing all the people who loved me.

The process of releasing fear took time. I knew what anger and fear were all about; I was less familiar with peace and love. Even though I had begun to sense the possibility of change, I chose the familiar over the positive for some time to come. I continued to be immobilized by the idea of telling people that I was angry or wanted to do something differently. And the more I avoided confronting my feelings, the more angry people seemed to gather around me, and the more anger I felt. Through the slow process of dealing with my feelings in the safety of my psychiatrist's office, my terror attacks began to subside.

Biofeedback and Control

At some point during that same year, I began biofeedback training. That process taught me how to modify the physical responses that were increasing my discomfort. I was evaluated in three main areas: body temperature, sweat reflex, and muscle tension. Two of those areas were of immediate concern.

When I was in pain, my body temperature went down. Over time, I learned how to control that response and keep my temperature close to normal. Another response to pain was the tensing of my face, neck, shoulders, and upper back muscles. I practiced relaxing those areas as a machine beeped to remind me when I fell back into my old pattern.

Learning more about my reactions to pain was helpful. I learned to control my responses when the machine was there to remind me, but it was not easy to maintain control when the beeps were gone. I used relaxation tapes at home to help with the transition, but so much was happening that it was hard for me to maintain composure even under the best of circumstances. It took many years of practice before I was able to relax my body quickly and easily.

Just as my Alexander Technique teacher had shown me how to hold my body and move in ways that would create less pain and discomfort, biofeedback gave me an internal gauge for measuring the responses that also increased my pain. Comparing the two techniques and the various physical responses they addressed made me more fully aware of the insidiousness of my disease.

Rheumatoid Arthritis meant so much more than the destruction of my joints. It affected most parts of my body and most of its functions. As a person who always wanted to know the why and how of everything, I wondered where all these problems had come from—had they always been tucked away inside me? Had the disease brought on all this turmoil? I realized that asking these questions, as natural as they felt, was a waste of time. The fact was that the problems existed, and I needed to deal with them as they were. The more time I spent wondering why, which in my case meant trying to find people to blame, the more time I wasted.

Back to the O.R.

Although I understood this, I still brooded over the "extras" or unexpected traumas that I had been forced to deal with since the onset of this disease. Adding them up, I realized what the cycle of illness was teaching me: The next trauma was never far behind.

I had finally admitted that the surgery on my index finger had failed, and that my pinky was useless. I was also tired of having a wrist and hand that looked like something from the twilight zone, so I went back to the surgeon to ask his opinion about trying again. He recommended replacing all the major joints in the hand; they were going anyway. And while he was at it, he could fix up the wrist by shaving off some bone and remodeling it.

I scheduled surgery and waited, with plenty of time to get nervous. It seemed that the more I tried to force myself to relax, the more tense I became. Being able to relax was not one of my strong points and I didn't understand that I couldn't force myself to be calm. It would take more than two weeks of practice to relax a body that had been in battle position for 29 years. As the date for surgery drew near, I realized that this one was the big time—four new joints and a new wrist.

Again, I did not have general anesthesia—just a partial block and a lot of valium. As I was rolled into the operating room, the surgeon asked if I would like to watch the procedure. At that moment I knew why they told me not to eat after midnight the day before the operation. If there had been anything in my stomach, I would have vomited all over him. As he showed me the little saw he would use to cut away the bone, switching it on and off, I began to think that maybe this surgery wasn't such a bright idea.

It wasn't.

The recuperation period was a little easier this time, if only because I knew what to expect. The need to ask other people for help continued to cause intense inner turmoil, at home and at work. As a matter of fact, just about everything was the same with this second surgery, including the lack of follow-up occupational or physical therapy.

I did exercise by myself at home, to the point of pain. Hoping that maybe a physical or occupational therapist could push me much further, I asked the surgeon about it. He said he did not believe that PT or OT would help. Feeling angry but powerless, I dropped the subject.

Lots of Pain, No Gain

Two months later I again faced the reality that my tendons were stuck. Now all four joints of my right hand were immobile. My hand was a badly carved piece of wood. The only movement came from the middle joints in the fingers, except the pinky, which was already useless from the first surgery. Because my thumb did all the work for my hand, it was constantly swollen, red, and sore.

It's difficult to say how I felt when I realized that both operations had been failures. When I try to remember my feelings, all I see is a blank screen. I mentally checked out for a while, refusing to deal with the situation. Finally I came back to reality enough to realize that the results of the second surgery justified my feelings of open rage. After the first surgery, even though I was angry, at least I had relief from constant pain.

At that point, I switched to a new method of approaching life.I made an appointment with another rheumatologist for a second opinion about my treatment. Openly hostile to the surgeon, I stopped going for follow-up visits. My rage grew out of control, attacking anyone who crossed my path, unleashing bursts of hate that reverberated through my body as intense pain. The more I lashed out, the more I hurt.

I began to experience physical agony in places on my body that I never even knew existed. All the tendons and muscles up and down my legs signalled hot, angry pain. Each movement became an expression of the anger, guilt, and hatred I felt. Mentally I just wanted to hide, to stay in my room and sleep. My body cooperated fully by refusing to allow me to move, and I eliminated all but the most necessary activities from my life.

I continued to go to therapy, work on the Alexander Techniques, and see my rheumatologist. I got gold shots, not because they were helping, because they seemed to be my only hope. The second rheumatologist I saw reached the same conclusion—he recommended that I continue the treatment I was already receiving. But no matter how hopeless I felt, a spark inside continued to prompt me, "keep going, find another way."

At that point, a member of my family suggested that I apply to a pioneering research facility in the area. Maybe they could suggest some other alternatives. I asked my doctor for a reference. He didn't believe that my case fit their research needs, but he agreed that I should give it a try.

Even my desire to try something new left me afraid and guilty. I had strong faith in my doctor, and I knew he had given me all he had. Even though our communication was not great, I knew that he wanted the best for me. Fighting the disease together all those years, we had developed a relationship based on mutual respect, and on my part, sheer need. But the reality of the situation had begun to fester inside me. Despite years of care from a good doctor, a fine representative of the medical establishment, I was unable to walk without tremendous effort. I had gone through two major operations that could only be described as disastrous.

Who had failed? Me? The doctors? Were my expectations unrealistic? I had no idea what any of us had expected, because we had never taken the time to discuss the purpose—the final goals of my treatment. This vagueness began to make me feel extremely uncomfortable, and again I was shocked at how I had let my life drift. But something positive grew out of that discomfort. My desire to reevaluate what I was doing and explore alternatives was stronger than ever. Maybe I would find something that would lead me to a better reality than the one I was living.

VIII. EXPLORING ALTERNATIVES

Today, I don't believe that doctors were responsible for the progression of my disease. But five years ago, I blamed the entire medical profession for everything that had gone wrong. First, I was badly diagnosed. For the next six years, even after an accurate diagnosis, I got worse. I agonized through my twenties, in and out of doctor's offices, in and out of surgery. Rheumatoid arthritis probably would not have taken my life, but neither would it respond to medication like other diseases. One way to deal with an illness that lasts a lifetime is to find a series of people to blame. That was my pattern, but it only aggravated the problem. For me, blame was anger, and it turned inward to cause me one physical symptom after another.

In a search for solutions I was desperate enough to start therapy, develop a suicide pact, make a list, and start working on it. The list became urgently important as I sought to replace the men in white jackets who had molded my life since I was seven. But even as I pursued alternatives to traditional medicine, I was honest with myself on one point: I wanted to investigate the alternatives, but I still needed to see my doctor. His presence in my life was essential. I was ready, however, to decide exactly what role I wanted him to play.

What wasn't clear was why I had so freely consented in the past to treatments I wasn't sure of, but I did know that pain and fear were good reasons for holding on. The fear was that if I didn't do what the doctor said, I would become a hopeless cripple. At the same time, it was obvious that all my medical care so far had been ineffective. Given these two opposing beliefs, it no longer surprised me that nothing worked. How could anyone help a person whose own belief systems were at war? Clearly, I needed to ask myself a lot of questions.

Defining the Problem

First of all, how, for my purposes, could I define the word "doctor?" It seemed clear that my own doctor was an individual who saw his job as helping me live comfortably with the illness I had. If healing had occurred, he would have accepted it as luck, fate, or a temporary remission. Rheumatoid arthritis was not an illness most doctors would discuss in terms of healing. Because of this, at some level we all acknowledged defeat before we started.

The next question rocked me to the core: If what I believed about my doctor was true, did it not follow that by accepting his treatment I was an active participant in keeping the disease alive? How could it possibly be helpful to trust people who did not believe I could get well? Most importantly, did I believe that I could heal? Did I want to?

I asked myself what I really wanted—at that moment. It didn't matter what I had wanted when I was 19 or 21 or 25—or what I could realistically expect based on common theories about the possibility of curing RA. It quickly became clear that I didn't want to learn to live with this disease, or to get a little better. I wanted to live a disease-free existence. I wanted to beat the odds and erase this disease from my system.

After admitting that I really wanted to be a healthy person, I panicked for about two weeks. I had never before allowed myself the luxury of such an idea. Always before, when stray thoughts of healing popped into my head, I would ridicule myself for dreaming of achieving the impossible.

The next question that needed an answer was, "Did I want to believe that, with help, I could be cured?" My answer, of course, was yes, but I was plagued by doubts and had no faith to fall back on—only a gut feeling that maybe I could find the faith somewhere. Connected to that was another question: Could my desire for health be reconciled with my doctor's approach to my disease, and if so, how? Could we possibly continue to work as a team?

The most important question dealt with my own power to change. How could I exchange my tired old convictions for vigorous new ones? Clearly they were not the same, and I knew that unconscious doubts were holding me back. Because I had been unwilling to claim and fight for my beliefs, the only ones I could work with were those of the people around me. Now that I wanted to decide who I was, I wasn't sure how to do it.

Dealing with the Doctor

When I felt strong enough, I began to share my thoughts and questions with my doctor, only to find that we didn't agree on much of anything. I continued to receive the gold shots, but I also moved forward with the other items on my list.

Acknowledging my fear when it began to seem overpowering somehow lessened its effect on my life. I kept my doctor informed as I tried each new form of treatment and he gave me as much support as he could, but our relationship was not the same. He was no longer my only hope; I was looking elsewhere with new determination. Years later I realized that the only thing I had ever really wanted from him was love, and that he had given me freely.

Making a first conscious statement of what I wanted, as opposed to what I believed, marked another difference in the way I viewed my life.

For someone who was into blaming other people for her problems, it was not an easy step to take. What if I tried every method on my list, and nothing worked? What if failed to make any basic changes in my beliefs? Who could I blame?

I didn't like the answer to that question, although I knew it would have been the same no matter when I had chosen to ask it. No one could cure me of problems that had to be healed from within. Other people could give me help, comfort, support, and medication to ease the pain, but control of my life had always been up to me.

I got very busy taking care of myself, getting involved with several things at the same time. I began group therapy and acupuncture treatments. My case had been accepted for review by doctors in the research facility, so I started making regular visits there. I began taking antidepressants to help ease the chronic pain that was keeping me awake, as well as because I was finally ready to admit that I was severely depressed. It would be nice to say that this new surge of activity meant I was off and running, but at least I was limping.

Just Me and My Group

Group therapy was difficult for me because I was uncomfortable with any kind of open interaction. In my world, people conspired with one another, on a one-to-one basis, against another person or group of people designated more or less temporarily as the enemy. In the past, I had managed to pair up with enough people so that I could identify almost everyone as the enemy.

But in this new group, my habit of constantly finding someone to complain about slammed me right in the face. Here was a whole crowd of people sitting right in front of me every week. No matter how awful, or insensitive, or disagreeable I found them, it was impossible to talk about any of them behind their backs. If for any reason someone missed a session, the conversation might tend to focus on the missing person. But the next week the story was always told. I couldn't even talk about the people in group during individual therapy; my psychiatrist wouldn't let me. The bottom line was that for the first time, I was being held accountable for what I said. The situation made me extremely uncomfortable. With my normal mode of operation unavailable, I didn't know how to act.

Once again, I found refuge in anger. I got mad at individuals in the group and at the group as a whole. The protection of the group allowed me to express anger with my psychiatrist in a way I had never permitted myself before. Other group members became angry with me. Two or more of us would join forces and become collectively angry at someone else within or outside the group. And despite all of our shared problems, we managed to work out a good deal of our rage.

Occasionally, members of the group would become intensely emotional—crying openly for long periods of time. Dealing with this left me not only exhausted, but jealous. I was torn between trying to get them to stop and wanting to join them. Crying (or not allowing myself to cry) was an ongoing issue for me.

Working with a group made me realize how much of myself was locked up inside, made me see that it was important to take off the mask and reveal who I was. It became even clearer that for all the years I thought I was shielding other people with my silence, I had only been protecting myself and my inability to deal with feelings. It became important to find a way to form opinions and state them rationally and peacefully. Along with that process, I had to learn to set limits on what I would tolerate from other people.

After two years in group therapy, I came to understand that it didn't matter who I was dealing with or what his or her age: I was deserving of respect. I recognized that I attracted and was drawn to people with very strong personalities, and because I was unable to set limits, I allowed them to bully me. As a matter of fact, I seemed to enjoy letting people abuse me so that I could complain about being mistreated. Such fun to play the martyr!

Group therapy also showed me the flip side of my reluctance to acknowledge or tolerate my own feelings: I also resisted allowing others to express their feelings. My usual response to emotional discussions was to show physical discomfort and try to shut them up. It was difficult, but I started working on letting others express themselves without allowing my own discomfort to interfere.

My real desire to change was a good start. Another struggle was to keep myself out of situations in which I could become the martyr. I learned that it was essential to take a deeper look at situations that made me uncomfortable, although I still avoided doing so whenever possible. Feelings of peace and relaxation were so threatening that I usually managed to create chaos and the familiar feelings that I had previously accepted as normal.

At the same time, I realized that I tended to give and receive love in self-destructive ways—ways that contributed significantly to my chronic illness. To save my body, I had to relearn what it meant to love and care for myself and other people. The biggest issue here was to learn that it was possible to say no in a loving manner, then to follow through on it. Consciously, I knew what constituted a good relationship. But I had many unconscious beliefs that had to be confronted and released before I could actually have what I said I wanted.

Joining the therapy group was part of my unspoken commitment to resolve the inharmonious relationships in which I constantly found myself. Even though I became sicker during this period than I had ever been before, the group experience was essential to my healing. That group set in motion a process of self- confrontation that would continue to transform my life.

Adventures in Acupuncture

The acupuncture experiment resulted from desperation—I was feeling so bad that anything was worth a try. After making the first appointment, I realized that I knew nothing about the process except that some friends had seen it help people with a variety of ailments, including RA. When I discussed acupuncture with my rheumatologist, he said that it sometimes seemed to help RA, but that the results tended to be temporary. His patients who had tried acupuncture had to go back again and again to continue feeling well.

Hey, no problem! I had been going to doctors for eight years with little or no benefit. His opinion wasn't designed to encourage me, but it did. Even for minimal results, I was perfectly willing to get one treatment a day for the rest of my life.

But as the time came for my first appointment, I began to have doubts. I was already spending every cent and every spare second chasing health from office to office, city to city, and I had never felt worse. Did I really need to set up one more weekly activity? Five years later I would see how each part of the process helped, but while I was in the middle of it and still feeling horrible, none of it made much sense. In the end, I decided to give it a try. If nothing spectacular happened, I didn't have to go back.

Pulling up for my appointment, I was put off by the fact that the acupuncturist's office was in his home. Although I had known this from the start, it was one more reason to drag my feet. I never liked keeping appointments, business or medical, in anyone's home. There were enough cooking odors in my own house; I had no desire for anyone else's. It was important for me to see people in neat little offices so that I didn't have deal with their attachments or life styles. I almost turned around and drove off, but again, something inside told me to stay and see it through.

The results of the acupuncture were spectacular from the very first treatment. But I found that like everything else I was involved in, acupuncture was a process that required commitment. How sad to think that if I had not been deeply impressed by my first treatment, I would have missed another part of my healing experience.

For as long as I could remember, I had not perspired. I had taken it for granted, believing that it was the way my body worked, or didn't work.

After quizzing me about each and every bodily function I could possibly want or need in life, Bob inserted a few needles into the top of my back between my shoulder blades and let them sit there for a while. As I rolled my eyes and silently categorized this as not only unpleasant but another waste of time, a flood broke loose. Water began to seep from my underarms and every pore. Soon I had to ask for a towel. Enough perspiration drained out of me during that hour to make up for the 20 years I had been dry. As I made my next appointment, my feelings ran the gamut from embarrassment to wonder. Exhausted, I drove home and collapsed.

The acupuncture process helped me get my body, mind, and spirit in order—or balance—with the elements inside and around me. I became more aware of how my body and mind reacted to seasonal changes, to various foods, to being generally out of alignment. During each treatment, I asked Bob what "we" were working on this week, and he would explain. Sometimes I listened; sometimes I didn't. I was not well versed in yin and yang, but then I didn't have to be. I believed that these treatments were going to help me whatever the state of my ignorance, and I knew how quickly the process could work. My first experience was proof.

Bob was the first person to ask out loud a question that had been tormenting me for months: Why was I getting the gold shots? What did I hope to accomplish by continuing to take them years after they had proven to be a waste of time and money? He was also the first person I told that I was still getting them because I was afraid not to—that there was no sane reason why I continued with what appeared to be useless treatments.

He also said something else that had been lurking in the back of my mind: there was no way for the injected gold to leave my body. I was dealing with a substance that had the capacity to be toxic, as my rashes, sores, and itching had shown. He believed that the longer I took gold, the longer it would take me to heal. I was pitting two forces against each other, allowing my body to be the battleground. He also told me that in England, the use of gold treatments was being seriously questioned by the medical profession.

Bob never lectured me, only told me how he felt about what I was doing. He understood my reluctance to break away from the medical establishment, but he also knew that I was moving in the direction of doing so. I was able to tell Bob that I was not yet willing to stop seeing my doctor. For many years, he had been the only person I felt I could turn to, and I was attached to him not only as a physician, but as a person. I had called him in the middle of the night from places all over the country and he had always taken my calls. He was someone who understood, as well as a healthy man could, what I was going through. But I did consciously begin the mental process of releasing myself from his care.

By far the most important element about my acupuncture treatments was the releasing of fluids, not only perspiration, but tears. And it wasn't just the acupuncture that helped me cry—as in a jigsaw puzzle, each piece of what I was doing was linked to the next. But I do believe that acupuncture was one of the main forces behind my growing desire to cry.

I had been receiving treatments for a few months and had found myself able to let out more and more of my feelings. Then one day, Bob told me that he was going to balance my water element. I said fine and thought nothing of it. Before I knew it I was crying uncontrollably. Up until then, crying had meant one or two tiny drops of fluid. I was furious because, in my book, crying still meant loss of control. I remember screaming at him that he knew how much crying embarrassed me—he had done this on purpose and I would never forgive him.

I refused to make another appointment, and as I raced out the door I told him I would never see him again as long as I lived. I cried all the way home and didn't stop for what seemed like days. After a while, I was able to understand how significant this was and that it represented progress. Of course I went back, but that was the angriest time in my whole healing saga.

During the same period, I had been working in therapy to resolve my conviction that the way to solve a problem was not to acknowledge it, never speak of it again, never go back, never forgive. In practice, when things went wrong, I would simply leave. It took tremendous effort for me to call Bob and make another appointment, but I did. By now I was learning lessons by the minute and making changes where I had never thought I could. But physically, I was feeling more pitiful than ever.

The Yak Dung Caper

Going for acupuncture treatments led me to another adventure in healing, this time to New York City and the personal physician to the Dalai Lama. At Bob's suggestion, I made an appointment with the Lama's doctor on one of his rare visits to the United States. It may have been my first real step into activities that many would call weird, but by that time I was feeling so bad that each step took 20 minutes of effort.

Getting around in New York City wasn't easy, but I had a mission.

My friend and I arrived at the address in Manhattan to find a line of waiting people that went down five stories, out the door, and on to the street. We inched along for a few hours and were finally inside. An aide told me to urinate in a plastic container and take it in to the doctor. When I saw him take a taste of my urine, I was so impressed I would have done anything he said.

He looked at my hands and asked me through an interpreter not to have any more plastic put in my body. He explained to me that there were other ways to get well; that I needed to be patient. Finally he wrote out a long and complicated prescription with instructions about when and how to take it. His aide gave me my first supply of the "pills," which looked like brown and black pebbles of different sizes. Some had to be kept in the dark; some were to be taken on an empty stomach—there were all kinds of instructions. The trickiest part was that I had to send to Tibet for refills, but that didn't seem like a big deal.

So I started taking them. When people asked me what it was, I would always reply, "yak dung." It made them laugh and they stopped bothering me. I fully intended to continue with the yak dung for one year. The doctor had guaranteed that if I did, I would get well. But some complications arose that prematurely ended the treatments.

First of all, I was still taking anti-depressants. I discussed the yak dung with my psychiatrist. He was somewhat uneasy at the fact that I didn't know what was in it, but he was also a good sport who knew that if I believed in something strongly enough, it just might work. He gave a hesitant okay, knowing that I was going to take them no matter what anyone said. How could he argue? I was sure those pills could heal me in one year, as promised. My rheumatologist was amused by this new twist; he just smiled and wrote on my chart that I was taking yak dung daily until further notice.

Things went pretty well for a while, but then I raised my dose of anti-depressants and began hallucinating. If I didn't take the yak dung and the anti-depressants on the same day, I didn't hallucinate. Taking the two of them together at a high dose, however, was another story.

Occasionally I would call my psychiatrist to tell him my face was falling off, or the skin on my legs was melting, or my nose was misplaced. I was constantly losing and finding body parts. One good thing about all the confusion was that I didn't have a lot of time to think about pain—I was too busy trying to find my face.

One day when I managed to calm down enough for a sane chat with my psychiatrist, he told me I had to make a choice—either stop the anti-depressants or the yak dung (by now everyone was calling it yak dung). One or the other had to go—he would support my choice, whatever it was. It was the first time he had given me an ultimatum like that and I took it seriously. I was also struck by the fact that he did not say the yak dung had to go; he never told me it was ridiculous to take it.

About that same time, civil war broke out in Tibet. I had been receiving regular shipments of pills once a month. At the time when I was deepest into the hallucinations, the monthly shipment didn't arrive.

Even if it had arrived, I would probably have stopped taking yak dung anyway. The deciding factor would have been that it didn't help me sleep and the anti-depressants did. I needed sleep, partly to keep me out of misery for as many hours of the day as possible. I must say that I missed the hallucinations. They had become a fun diversion. They didn't scare me, although I was having some trouble functioning and interacting in the real world.

Dealing with Change

At this point, one might reasonably ask how I managed to do my job. Frankly, I'm not sure. I remember going to work and keeping busy, but I couldn't have been giving it my all. That part of the story was nothing new. The only thing I had ever really devoted myself to was being sick. By this time, thanks to some very supportive administrators and a note from my doctor, I was out of the classroom and writing. Doing paperwork while hallucinating was much easier than trying to work with teenagers.

I also have no idea how I managed to come out of that period with any friends. As I became busier and busier with healing, I had no time for anyone or anything except work, appointments, and sleep. The pain was so bad that if I did make social plans, I almost always cancelled them. But most of my friends stood by me even though they might not have understood what I was doing. It's not often that someone disappears for three years and I'm sure that some people still wonder where I went.

Of course there were others who did not like the changes I was making. Some of my friends became defensive, thinking that because I was changing, they would have to change, too. Some fell through the cracks when we couldn't find any way to mesh the "new me" with the "old them." But new friends appeared who were able to accept me and my struggle to build a new life, and to support and encourage me through even more changes.

By this time, I was at the half-way mark. Two and a half years had passed since I had written the list and entered the pact. During those years, I had finally allowed myself not only to ask for help, but to seek it actively. I had changed from a woman who passively accepted whatever happened to one who was purposefully involved in seeking ways to heal. I was beginning to believe that the choices I had written on that piece of paper were as readily available to me as to anyone else—that maybe I was more worthy than I had originally thought.

More importantly, something was beginning to happen inside me. I felt a letting go—a giving way of my spirit of doom. Of course the process of letting go met tremendous resistance from the part of me that was comfortable in my old way of life. The more I learned to trust and to accept help, the sicker I got. I also continued to believe that things would get worse before they got better, and this time, I was right.

The sicker I got the more determined I was to see my pact through to the end—I would not reevaluate anything until the entire five years were up. I was fiercely stubborn about this. My desire to live had begun to assert itself. Occasional thoughts of suicide were still very strong, but in spite of all the pain, they came to me less and less often.

IX. FIGHTING BACK

The reviewing physicians at the research facility had called me for an evaluation meeting. I would need to be there for one full day. My frame of mind was not good when I walked into the building that morning, and it got worse as the day went on. I went through the motions of being a patient, barely polite and staring at the clock.

Once again, I had blood taken, X-rays, physical exams—the regular medical routine. The results of the tests wouldn't give any new information—I knew that. I was so tired of the standard approach that I was literally sick on and off throughout the day.

Late in the afternoon, I met with the doctors. As I sat down, I sized up these people who were prepared to give me their expert opinions of my physical fate. Because of my long experience with doctors, I was able to sort out the interns immediately. That was important. With so many doctors around I needed a quick way to decide who I really had to deal with and who I could ignore. As it turned out, I only needed to be concerned with one.

Another Small Rejection

As the doctor started talking I found myself almost in a trance. He told me my case didn't fit their research needs; the reasons for that decision sailed right past me. I wasn't sure what he was talking about and really didn't care; this was one rejection I could handle. I had no desire to be involved in research projects that required me to take experimental drugs. What I did want was information on possible alternatives to what I was already doing. After he finished with his summary, I asked the doctor if he had any ideas to give me. He said no—that all he would suggest was to continue with the treatment prescribed by my current physician and increase the amount of gold I was taking.

He went on to indicate that he was somewhat surprised that I had applied there, that I wasn't as sick as most people who were referred. The only thing he could do was refer me to the occupational and physical therapy units (OT and PT) at the facility because of the total immobility in the joints of my right hand.

As those words reverberated through my skull, I felt an explosion of rage and the dawn of a new fantasy. I saw myself picking up a rifle I had hidden under the table and blowing him away—then turning to each staff member present and doing the same.

That fantasy gave me such pleasure that I began to use it often. I even investigated buying a gun and taking shooting lessons, but didn't follow through because I honestly felt I was dangerous. As it was, my bottled up anger was emerging in blasts and I felt very unstable. I realized I was one person who should not be walking around with a gun and the knowledge of how to use it.

Anyway, I finally lost my composure and went on a verbal rampage. I told him he should really think about the things he said to people. I, for instance, was quickly losing the ability to care for myself physically, and was just learning how to deal with rage. He had no idea what I had been through: to him I represented a piece of paper—a file that might possibly fit the needs of one of his projects. I was outraged at his lack of sensitivity: he was just one more person who didn't understand that I was looking for some good reasons not to kill myself.

I proceeded to tell the doctor and everyone else within earshot that he—in his glorious state of health and power—had no right to impose his judgement of how sick I was on me and my body. How dare anyone tell me I wasn't sick enough to be there. I had spent 30 years being sick—I was the expert here!!

Furthermore, I was there specifically to prevent myself from reaching his criteria of being sick enough, to keep myself from ever meeting the needs of any of his damn research projects. I stormed out of the room and spent the next hour looking for my car—in the maze of parking levels I couldn't remember where I had left it. This was another blessing in disguise. Driving in the state I was in, I might have run over the first jogger I saw without one regret. By the time I found the car, I was so exhausted I could barely turn the key to unlock the door.

Meeting the Folks in OT/PT

As it turned out, referral to the OT/PT unit was the best thing that doctor could have done for me. Before that fateful meeting I had decided that my goal and reward for subjecting myself to another round of tests would be to find one new alternative. Against all odds, his referral turned out to be exactly what I wanted. Even better, the treatments he suggested were already on my list. Later I was awed at how perfectly the situation had worked out. But during my meeting with the doctors, all I had really heard was one statement:

"You aren't as sick as most people who are referred."

I didn't hear from the Occupational or Physical Therapy Units for a long time—several months. When I did, I was reluctant to set up an appointment because that meant I had to subject myself to another physical examination. But OT and PT were on my list, and here was my chance to see if they would help.

Thinking about OT and PT reminded me of several good reasons to be angry. 1) I could not use my hand, even after all that surgery. 2) The surgeon who was supposed to have helped me had only succeeded in imposing his distrust of OT and PT on me. 3) Again, I had failed to speak up for what I felt I needed. I thought I had forgotten about all that, but realized it was only buried slightly below the surface.

I decided to make the appointment and keep it—letting anger get in the way would only hurt me. About three weeks later, I found myself in the middle of another physical exam given by the head of the OT/PT unit and about five interns. On my way out, I overheard her tell the interns to watch how I moved so that they would be aware of the typical "RA walk." It would have been more tactful for her to alert them before I came in, but I decided I might as well get used to being treated like a lab specimen.

As I left, someone told me that I would be contacted if they could be of service. Two weeks later, one of the occupational therapists called to set up a time to meet and discuss therapy. I was still upset, but my desire to try OT overwhelmed the self-destructive urge to say no. I made the appointment and went.

Bonnie (the therapist) took one look at my hand and went through the ceiling. She was furious that I had not had follow-up therapy, especially since both sessions of surgery had resulted in failure. I really enjoyed her rage—she expressed it even better than I could. And I was grateful at finding someone else who felt I had a right to use my hands.

Bonnie wanted to work with me three times a week, which was impossible because of my already packed schedule. We settled on once or twice a week, depending on how often I could get there. She expressed tremendous concern that I couldn't come more often, but I was literally running out of time.

She also managed to get me to agree to meet with the surgeon from a nearby teaching hospital under the guise of needing his opinion about what to do with my hand. Just hearing the word "surgeon" put me in a panic. But the appointment wasn't for another month—I had plenty of time to change my mind. At the time I made the appointment, I had absolutely no intention of going.

I hadn't grasped the intensity of the time commitments I had made. My schedule was truly outrageous, and I was in so much pain that I was no longer really walking. I shuffled my feet, never picking them off the ground unless I had to. As I moved, I hugged walls and railings for support. I was working full-time, going to individual and group therapy, getting acupuncture treatments and gold shots, taking lessons on the Alexander Technique, and now I had agreed to show up for OT once or twice a week. Something had to give, and I decided it would be the Alexander Technique. I had spent more than six months learning about it. I had the basic principles down and needed to work on carryover, but was losing my motivation to go because it hurt too much to move. It was hard to follow through on my decision to stop, because I was afraid that if I did, I would get worse.

Mistrusting my own judgement, I would have felt much better if my Alexander teacher had told me she thought I was ready to go out on my own. Of course, she couldn't do that—any decision about ending the work was up to me. But soon I was so busy with my new schedule that I forgot all about the trauma of that decision.

I always looked forward to my occupational therapy appointments. For one thing, Bonnie taught me how to use devices that made everyday living much easier. It was an incredible relief to find ways to get more use out of a hand that had become a liability.

Each time I shuffled into the OT unit, I found myself dealing with anger again. Why hadn't anyone told me about this equipment before? Why hadn't I asked? Opening jars and bottles had become almost impossible, but not with the new devices Bonnie showed me. Why had I spent so many years in the dark?

Surgery? Why, Of Course!

Before I knew it, it was time to see the surgeon. I found myself torn between wanting to keep the appointment and hear his opinion and a desire to run the other way. One thing I knew was that if I didn't show up, I would still have to face my therapist. This realization brought with it the fantasy of not seeing her again, but I knew I'd go back. Not only was I getting a lot out of the sessions, I was still very much into approval. I wanted Bonnie to think I was good girl, and good girls keep their appointments. I was also sincerely curious about this surgeon. He obviously believed in OT and PT or he wouldn't be affiliated with the unit. What would he say? I kept the appointment.

As it turned out, he had plenty to say. He felt that he could increase the mobility of my joints by 50 to 75 percent by doing the whole procedure over. But after examining my left wrist, he felt that it couldn't support me through another surgery in its present state. In other words, in order to fix the right hand, he first had to fix the left one. "Fixing" the left hand, he assured me, meant only a little cleaning up and support for the wrist—the joints were okay.

We would follow up both operations with OT, as many times a week as I could get there. He wanted to schedule the first surgery as soon as possible and the second six months later. Wonderful!

No matter how confident and matter-of-fact he sounded, I wasn't ready to hear any of it. I'm still amazed that I sat through his speech, but one thing he said held my attention: 50 to 75 percent more mobility. Compared with the zero mobility I had at that point, 50 to 75 percent was an offer I couldn't refuse.

Lately, my left wrist had taken incredible abuse. It was swollen, made snapping noises, and hurt badly enough to keep me awake nights. It was now the primary support for any activity that depended on my hands, which was almost everything I did. If I wanted to keep it working, it needed extensive repairs. As I listened to the surgeon, I knew I couldn't continue to ignore what had happened to my hands without paying an even higher price later.

After we talked for a while, I told the surgeon how happy I was that he believed in OT and PT. He took my hands gently and said that he had been a surgeon for a long time and honestly wasn't sure what he believed. He told me the one thing he was sure of was that I deserved to get more out of my hands and that he would do everything in his power to see that I did. His concern and honesty made me feel that I had found the right person to do the job.

Leaving the building, I began to feel callous. How could I deal with my body as if it were a washing machine in need of new parts? It had become a matter of deciding how long the left wrist could last until I needed surgery, and what could be done to put off that surgery as long as possible. I was beginning to see my body not as something that was generally in good working condition and needing minor, infrequent repairs, but as a mechanism in constant disorder, a constant candidate for crisis intervention. My days had become filled with the game of finding ways to do as much as possible between service calls.

Surgery? Oh, No!

So for the third time in less than two years, I signed up for surgery. I had a month to wait for the first operation and seven months for the second. I really hadn't had much time to think before my first two operations; the decision to act had been close to the actual dates. The third surgery was not too far off, but something about that fourth one bothered me. The idea of waiting around for seven months with the knife hanging over my head left me severely depressed. Thoughts of that fourth operation cast a shadow over my existence—I felt that I was on death row waiting to be executed.

For the next seven months, I experienced more pain than I had ever known, took more pills than I thought it was possible to swallow, and slept more than I was awake. I shuffled through each day like a zombie, so deeply drugged that I didn't care about anything except getting back to bed.

Entering pre-op one month later, I had to be helped onto the operating table because I couldn't lift my own body. My five- foot, eight-inch body weighed 100 pounds. My shoulders sagged and my head felt like dead weight. Glancing at my reflection in the mirror, I saw that I had the posture of a 95 year-old- woman. I didn't have enough muscle tone to lift my arm from my side, and if I had, the pain would have stopped me.

When I awoke, I remember feeling glad that at least the first part of this was over—now I only had a six-month wait. As I came to in the recovery room, several doctors came in to tell me that I was a wonderful patient. The anesthesiologist actually came over to show me pictures of his children; apparently I had asked to see them during surgery. I guess I was much more cordial on valium. Once I thought about it, it was not unlike me to act like a guest at a tea party in the middle of surgery. I'm sure very few people knew the depths of my depression, but this brave little soldier couldn't figure out who to follow once the battle was over.

I recovered from my third bout of surgery in a haze of drugs. The surgeon had poked around inside, given my tendon a "lift," and scraped away a lot of disease. I went home with a generous prescription of my favorite narcotic, Percocet, as happy as could be expected. And if the Percocet failed to keep me happy, I always had my anti-depressants.

With the left hand in a cast and my right hand immobile, I was forced to depend completely on other people. Although I didn't like it, this time I was grateful for the help because I truly could not do anything for myself. For anyone reading this book who has not been in that kind of situation, I will tell you that being totally dependent on others was the hardest lesson of my life.

There was no fooling myself this time. I was at the mercy of whoever was around and felt like taking care of me. The combination of pain, immobility, drugs, and depression left me useless. Because I lived through this experience and found a way to get well, I will never take anything or anyone for granted again. Any time I do start to fall back into my old patterns or feel ungrateful, one look at either of my hands brings me right back to where I need to be.

I didn't need a lot of occupational therapy for the left wrist. It was mobile when I went into surgery and he had done nothing to make it worse. My left elbow froze, however, and required a lot of attention before I could move it again. That was my first experience with the Physical Therapy Unit. Meanwhile, my OT instructor was continuing her efforts to get my right hand to do something—anything. The joints were fixed, and the tendons were stuck to the bones, but we worked with what we had.

Welcome to Now

Somehow, the time passed. About four months after surgery, the pain in my body began to subside. I was ecstatic but tortured by the fear that it would come back at the same level. It seemed that every time I turned around, there was a new lesson to learn.

One big lesson had to do with my habit of living in the past or the future, but never in the present. The great question I constantly asked myself was, "What will I do if what happened before happens again?" Dealing with that one allowed me to worry about the past and the future at the same time!! The present moment never had a chance to shine through as a healing experience. Only now, three years later, I'm able to see that time for what it was: the true beginning of my physical healing.

I continued with acupuncture, group and individual therapy, gold shots, and OT. Hesitantly, I began to live a little more, but was reluctant to do too much because I was afraid I'd get sick again. Gradually, I was able to decrease the amount of drugs I was taking. I was still in pain, but instead of hurting all the time, now I only hurt when I moved. I had even begun to put on some weight, and I had my hair cut professionally for the first time in almost two years.

X. THE CONCEALED ALTERNATIVE

One day I emerged from my drugged stupor and started to worry. It was more than three years since I had written the pact, and I seemed to be right back where I had started. Wasn't three years enough time to get well? For that matter, how could I define "well?" Should I base my decision on what I had recently lived through, or on the fact that I seemed to be back where I had started?

It had never occurred to me that it would be so difficult to decide whether or not I was well. I had written the pact with the concrete idea that people are either sick or healthy, and they know the difference. Now I was more aware of grey areas that needed to be considered, and not a little irritated at finding them.

Each morning I found myself counting days—how many until the next surgery, and how many since I had begun to feel better. As usual, I was reliving the past, dreading the future, and ignoring the present. As I became aware of the precious time I was wasting, I realized that killing time like this allowed me to kill myself figuratively without actually doing the deed. These moments would never come again— these days were gone forever. How could I look at the way I was living and justify my existence?

Sometime during this period of waiting I began to assume full responsibility for myself, and it gave me hope. If I was capable of making such a mess of my life, I was also capable of cleaning it up. The past was gone and the future had no meaning until it arrived. All I had to do was figure out a way to live happily in the present, but how could I learn to live in the only time that was real? The pain began to ease, became nothing more than physical discomfort. That told me two things: I had come a long way and I still had a long way to go. It also occurred to me that five years just might not be enough time to get well.

A New Kind of Freedom

The big day was coming. One way or another, my years of surgery were almost over. And I had more hope for good results from this surgery than I had held for any of the other three. But as usual, hope had its down side. What if, like the first two, this operation didn't work? What if I found myself sicker than before?

No matter how good I felt the first half of any given hour, my mood always found its way back to hopelessness by the hour's end. Conversely, if I started an hour in despair, it would end in hope. Two conflicting thoughts carried on a constant battle in my head: "I've had enough. I can't do this any more," and "If I can just get through this, I'll be okay."

Thoughts like these led me to do something that only a person truly unsure of life would do: I got a loaded gun and kept it under my bed—just in case this last surgery was unsuccessful. Of course, thinking seriously about suicide negated any attempt to face and change the barren reality I had created. I could never be fully committed to life as long as death remained such an attractive option. My doubts about the existence of God and the value of my life made freedom from pain seem a desirable consequence of suicide.

Still, the idea that I really could kill myself gave me an illusion of strength, despite my fears of going under the knife again. Death seemed the way to gain final control, not over other people, but over the physical pain that sucked movement and joy from my body. It tempted me as the ultimate form of freedom.

Knowing that this was not a typical definition of freedom made me reluctant to discuss my feelings about the future with anyone. Who wants to pal around with a woman whose most cherished fantasy is to wake up in the morning pain-free? Equating freedom with self-imposed death wasn't a very popular concept. The visions of freedom that other people described—of walking the beach whenever they wanted, having enough money to travel, living a life of leisure—were meaningless to me.

At that time, I often ate lunch with a close friend. We sometimes talked about being alone, compared ways to get through fears and bad moments. During one of those talks, my friend revealed that she kept a loaded gun near her bed. In fact, she actually had two guns. Driving home that night, I realized that I wanted the second one. I didn't consider the fact that I had no idea how to use it or that the weakness in my hands would make it almost impossible for me to lift it, let alone pull the trigger.

Of course I didn't tell my friend that I was contemplating suicide. Instead I lied, saying that my housemate was gone a lot and I was afraid to be alone. As we discussed my request, I could see that although she felt very uncomfortable, she understood what I was saying. She agreed to lend me the gun with the understanding that I would buy my own and give it back as soon as possible.

A few days later, she brought me the loaded gun in a brown paper bag. She handed it to me and we both looked around in panic. As I walked a few feet to put it away in my car, she drove off and another friend came into the parking lot. I must have looked guilty because he immediately asked me what was in the bag. The clown in me said, "Silly! It's a loaded gun," and I laughed as if he had just asked the most ridiculous question in the world. He laughed, too, and went on to his car. I unlocked my car door, put the gun under the seat, got in, and passed out.

When I came to, I thought to myself that anyone with half a brain would have told him it was a tuna sandwich and a soda. But no, I had to tell him the truth. The only good thing was that no one would have believed I was seriously contemplating suicide.

I drove home that afternoon feeling relaxed, visualizing the two possible scenarios. I would have this fourth surgery and if it worked, I would return the gun to my friend. If it didn't, I would take a pile of antidepressants and then blow my brains out. Driving along, I realized that the gun fantasies I had enjoyed at the medical facility were very close to becoming reality, except this time I would turn the gun on myself.

Surgery—Finale

Finally the big day arrived. I showed up at the hospital for my fourth operation in two and a half years, the third on my right hand. As I checked in, I wondered aloud if I was signing into the right kind of hospital. I went in feeling better physically and mentally than I had in months.

I sat in the waiting room, surrounded by others also scheduled for surgery. For a fleeting moment I wondered about these people—what were they thinking? Did they have as much pain as I? Soon I lost interest in them and my mind wandered back to the gun, my ticket to freedom, and to the friend who had unknowingly given it to me.

The receptionist's voice calling my name brought me back to reality. I filled out forms and answered questions, with nausea and an "oh-my-God-what-am-I-doing" panic running through me. In only six months I had forgotten how long it took for nurses with needles to find my skinny, squirmy veins. I had forgotten how scared I was when I went in and how sick I felt when I came out. I had forgotten how hospitals—all hospitals—smelled, and how long it took to recover. The only way I got through the morning was to keep reminding myself that it was almost over.

The doctor must have found a lot of work to do, because the surgery took a long time. Afterward, though it was extremely difficult to shake off the anesthesia, at least I knew he was finished. I was so worked up about this surgery that soon after I was rolled into my room, I began hallucinating that the doctor had forgotten to operate. I buzzed for the nurse. When she came in, I told her to get the doctor quickly—that he had forgotten to do the surgery and if he didn't do it that day, I wasn't coming back. She asked me to try to lift my right arm, turned me over, and gave me a shot of Demerol.

Three hours later I woke up and started the same routine. I spent the next nine hours sleeping, waking up, buzzing the nurse, and getting shots of Demerol. Each time I woke up, I screamed for the nurse to get the doctor, telling her that this was his last chance to fix my hand and that I couldn't believe he'd forgotten.

The nursing staff was very glad to see me discharged.

I began intensive occupational and physical therapy three or four days after the surgery, and it more than doubled the mobility in every joint. Because I could finally move, the swelling that had been present for two years went down, and my hand looked more "real" than I had ever thought it would again. Although it was nowhere near perfect, I was thrilled. I was also determined never to have surgery again.

The occupational therapist showed me how to hold and maneuver pans and cooking utensils to get the best use of my joints. She told me how much weight I could hold, and how to carry things that were difficult to grasp. To my delight and surprise, I found myself re-learning how to use my hand.

By the end of summer it was obvious that I was going to be all right. When I returned the gun to my friend, I finally told her the real reason I had borrowed it, and apologized for misleading her. As I suspected, she had never dreamed I was suicidal. She said that if I had used the gun, she would have felt like killing herself for giving it to me. It was shocking to realize that I had borrowed it without ever considering her feelings or her possible reaction to my death. My only concern had been for myself.

The occupational therapy continued through spring of the following year. When she was convinced that my hand was as mobile as she could get it, Bonnie waved me goodbye. Two or three months after the last surgery, I stopped taking both antidepressants and narcotics for pain. I did keep the leftover pills around, because I didn't trust my body to feel good for long.

The Vitamin Venture

All through this period, I had continued with group and individual therapy, as well as acupuncture. As I recovered from the fourth operation, I started to turn back to my list, but I didn't have time to decide which item to pursue next. Someone in my family had heard a radio show featuring a doctor who dealt with arthritis through vitamin therapy. She suggested that I see him. I made an appointment and off I went on what I thought was my next adventure in healing.

Driving to the nutritionist's office felt a lot like running—in circles. If I had started writing that day, the title of this book would have been "Linda Chases the Wind." As I drove, I imagined the wind touching my face, swirling around me—teasing me but never letting me touch. I had an impulse to grab the wind and hold it, but knew I couldn't possibly make a fist tight enough to hold the elusive stuff of my dreams: health.

Each night in dreams I found myself searching and searching but finding only part of what I needed—one sock of a pair; a dress with the belt missing; a car with the keys in the ignition but no gas. Nothing was whole. Waking or sleeping, I felt scattered and fragmented, with the missing pieces always just beyond my reach.

XI. CHASING THE WIND

Once again I managed to pull off my brave soldier act and keep the appointment at the nutrition clinic. By now I was totally disgusted with myself for gliding into this routine as if on automatic pilot, but when it was over, I always remembered who I was. I had the pain to thank for that.

I did realize that my negative feelings about this appointment had nothing to do with the way I felt about vitamins. Vitamin therapy and diet were two of the areas I intended to investigate. I vaguely understood that I was entering a new phase of my five-year plan, but I did not expect this to be the missing piece of the puzzle. I knew that it didn't matter how many vitamins I took or what kind of diet I went on—something was missing and until I figured out what it was, I wouldn't get well.

In order to have my visits to the nutritionist covered by insurance, I had to be examined by the staff M.D. With each new doctor, my annoyance grew. Why did they refuse to look at other recent test results, even if they were given for the same reasons? Before I went through with the tests, I tried to have the medical technician call some of my other doctors for the test results she needed. My attempts were unsuccessful, and I braced myself for the onslaught of needles, blood tests, urine tests, and the familiar and unforgettable smell of a medical lab. I left the office feeling wasted and desperate. I imagined the wind swirling around my feet, then vanishing forever.

I was exhausted—from the intensive OT, from the mental and physical strain of surgery, from subjecting myself to another medical workup, and from the realization that I had almost as much pain as I had almost three years earlier. Because there was nothing else to do, I waited for the test results.

A Pill for This, a Capsule for That...

My blood tests revealed mild allergies to certain foods and medications—some vegetables, fish, meats, grains, spices, fruits, nuts, dairy products. The only extreme allergy was to aspirin, but of course, I knew that. They told me to stay away from a short list of foods and condiments for six months, then gradually reintroduce them to my diet. I was to avoid aspirin as if my life depended on it.

The tests also indicated that only one of my T-cell counts was within normal limits. They prescribed a program of dietary supplements to battle this problem. A trace mineral analysis compared the concentration of specific minerals in my blood with "normal" levels. Many of the mineral counts were too high, possibly because of all the gold in my system. Again, supplements were prescribed. They had analyzed the amino acids in my system through both blood and urine tests. Again, I was in bad shape and in need of supplements.

Results of a test called the Heidelberg Gastrogram indicated that my stomach tended to "dump" food directly into my intestines without digesting it. In other words, I wasn't receiving much nutritional value from the food I was eating. This condition, along with the enormous quantities of drugs I had taken and my daily battles with stress, had left me unable to digest and use food the way most people did. More supplements were prescribed to remedy this "Stomach Dumping Syndrome."

The test I had tried hardest to resist was a "hair analysis." I had recently had a permanent, and knew that the test results would show me much closer to death than I actually was. I had also read that insurance companies usually refused to cover the cost of this test. The medical technician assured me that the test would give accurate results, and that it would be covered by insurance; both statements later proved to be untrue.

In this situation as in most others, my faltering self-esteem was constantly in the way. I found it impossible to say no and as the technician snipped off small wisps of hair, a lifetime of hostile subservience passed before me.

The combination of my inability to assert my own wishes and the dishonesty of the lab technician set up negative feelings between the nutritionist and me. Because of these feelings, I quit going for follow-up tests much earlier than I was supposed to, although I did continue taking the supplements.

As for the vitamins, by the time the total workup was done, I was taking approximately 50 different pills a day. It was a complicated routine—I had to take some before, some during, and some immediately after meals. Some were to be taken on an empty stomach, at least two hours after eating. It took a few weeks for me to get the schedule right, but soon I was keeping the supplements straight by color coding and size.

An even more difficult aspect of the routine was that I never stopped eating. I not only ate meals, I snacked constantly. Now, the instructions to take the supplements on an empty stomach meant I had to stop snacking, and I felt very deprived.

I followed the supplement regimen for two months and then went back for repeat testing. Almost everything had improved except mineral content—they found increased levels of mercury and aluminum in my blood, and prescribed more supplements to take care of that.

Although I was tired of explaining the many and varied facts of my medical treatments, it was difficult to hide the fact that I was taking 50 different kinds of supplements a day and had to alter my diet to do so. My supervisor at work was very kind and asked, "What are you taking now, dear?" She had lived through the yak dung experience with me, and nothing surprised her any more. Other people not so kind, began to tease me. I tried not to show how their well-meant jokes hurt my feelings; but for the first time, I did not allow my need for approval to stop me from doing what I wanted to do. I continued taking the supplements for almost a year. One day it suddenly seemed more trouble than it was worth to buy and take them, so I stopped.

Food, Glorious Food

A little while after I started on the supplements, I became more aware of what I was eating—and not eating. My usual diet was made up of a lot of meat, dairy products, and processed foods—generally anything fast and easy. While I knew that this was not the best diet for someone trying to get well, the job of investigating different nutritional approaches totally confused me.

There was no end of highly recommended diets, not only for general good health, but for arthritis. The Tibetan doctor had told me to avoid four foods: green peppers, pork, eggplant, and tomatoes. The nutritionist had asked me to avoid the foods on my allergy chart for six months, and as long as I took the supplements, anything else was fine. I wanted a more concrete plan to follow.

Collecting health and diet books, I realized wearily that I was going to have to do this on my own. A major investigation revealed total disagreement—even among those who should have been experts—about what people with rheumatoid arthritis should eat. I was tired of being presented with so many decisions. Why couldn't someone knock on my door, tell me exactly what to eat, and promise me immediate success?.

All my life I had been teased about skinniness (one popular nickname had been "bird legs"). With no weight problem, I had always eaten whatever I wanted and left dieting to other people. To me, a "diet" was simply a way to lose weight. As I continued with my research, I realized that the true meaning of diet had escaped me.

The first thing I did was chart everything I ate for a week. I was appalled. Although I had never really liked desserts, I routinely ingested large amounts of sugar through processed foods and sodas. I craved salt, and the fast foods I ate not only took care of that desire, they heightened it. Fresh vegetables rarely passed my lips, although I did eat fruit because it was easy and filling.

Both my sisters had been vegetarians for years. I had dismissed them as slightly fanatic, but it was true that the only time I ate well was with them. When I was alone, my old habits took over.

I began to question everything I ate and after much denial, I finally accepted the truth: like everything else, my diet reflected total lack of self-esteem. I didn't care enough about myself to eat well. I decided that it was time to change, but I couldn't imagine what I was going to eat. I continued to read, this time searching for healthy foods that sounded interesting.

Thinking that it would be easy to change my eating habits, I was in for a big surprise. It took me about seven months to change how and what I ate. Gradually I eliminated sodas, junk food, heavy spices, most dairy products, and sauces.

I did notice that when I was depressed, tired, or anxious, I went right back to my old eating habits. Although those were the times when I should have been the most careful, I ate junk. It's quite normal for people to identify certain foods with certain emotions and situations; I had just never realized that I did it. Soon it became clear that my diet would not stabilize until I did.

Macrobiotics and Me

At one point, I became interested in the macrobiotic system. I decided to try to follow a macrobiotic diet exclusively for six months—except for taking the supplements—to see if it would make a difference in how I felt. The foods for that diet included many that I had come to enjoy, so it wasn't difficult for me, except that I did miss eating raw fruit. I cut out all meat and added the types of fish that were recommended. Sugar was completely out.

The macrobiotic diet was very beneficial, giving my system a much-needed cleaning out. The best thing was that I had chosen the diet for myself and didn't feel deprived. When I found myself wanting other foods, I simply added them to my diet. My energy level went up, I was able to work harder and longer than before, I was no longer constipated, and the swelling in my joints went down significantly. Even my hair, thin and dull from years of medication, stress, and lack of vitamins, became healthier.

Gradually, I began feeling better. I know that the macrobiotic diet helped, along with all the other things I was doing. I continued to take acupuncture treatments and food supplements, and to participate in individual and group therapy. As I improved, physically and mentally, I felt confused about what to stop and what to continue. Two things I knew for certain: I was making some progress and I was very busy.

My experience with diets taught me that I had to deal with my eating habits as I did with anything else: it was my responsibility to be aware of what I ate and how it affected me. My diet was a choice that no one else could make for me. If I decided to eat poorly, I had only myself to blame for the consequences that would certainly follow.

XII. A TURNING POINT

Some time after the fourth operation and during the middle of my nutritional search, I had a major breakthrough.

Writing had always been my best method to express how I felt, but I never re-read or kept what I wrote—I wanted no permanent evidence of my true feelings. I had even stopped writing for a few months, when it got more and more difficult to throw my poems, essays, and stories away. This new conflict about throwing out my work scared me. If I kept the things I wrote, someone might read them and my secrets would be common knowledge. With that panicky thought in mind, I decided that it was much safer not to write anything at all.

But I could not handle this self-imposed exile from writing. It had been my surest path to emotional freedom. My need to express my feelings at least once before I trashed them was much stronger than I had realized.

As I continued the self-imposed ban on writing, my anger became so intense that I couldn't sleep, eat, or see straight. I felt like a bottled up mass of nerves, about to explode. For the first time, it was clear that this anger was literally hurting me. Equally obvious was the revelation that my anger was far greater than I had dreamed. I had reached those two crucial insights only because I had stopped writing. Without pinning my emotions down on paper, I had allowed them to run wild, finally demonstrating the full depth of the hatred that ran my life.

Writing *Letters to Mary*

The anger continued to grow until I thought I'd lose my mind. I craved the opportunity to share my feelings, knowing that it would ease the pain. But I didn't feel safe talking to anyone I knew. I needed someone special to direct my writing to—someone I knew I could trust—but someone who would not learn of the process until it was complete.

The only person I could think of was my older sister, Mary. She had taken care of me when I was sick and had done her best to love me in every way. She also lived in another state, and would be unlikely to drop in and find me working. But could I be honest with her?

One night, in sheer desperation, I sat down on my bed and started writing a letter to Mary. Hours passed as I poured out my feelings in a series of letters and poems. I wrote for days, deliriously happy to be expressing myself again. I didn't worry about whether to keep the work—I just kept writing. If I had known that some day I would consider making every word public, I might have jumped out the window.

The letters described everything I was going through and how I felt about it. As I wrote, I realized how badly I needed to leave anger and blame behind. I had found the missing link in the healing process—it was essential to find a way to express my anger, in order to let it go. If I could find a way to forgive, there would be room for love, and love would make me well.

Forgiving was the key to life in the present. Constantly rehashing anger and blame had kept me wallowing in the past for years. Seeking courage to say exactly what I felt, I worked hard not to censor myself because of guilt or a need for approval. The letters were full of bitterness, anger, and despair. Whether anyone ever saw them or not, writing them made me feel like a bad person. But I told myself not to worry about my failure to be a good girl—I'd have time to worry about that later.

I wrote constantly for about ten days and then stopped. A month or so later, I picked up the book again and wrote some more, sure that this time the story was finished. Two years later, this book is being written as one more extension of my letters to Mary. When I started writing *Letters to Mary* in 1985 (see appendix), I wasn't sure I'd be around for the ending.

Each time I finished each page of the manuscript, I kept it. It was the beginning of my search for a way to forgive. When I reread the pages, I realized that the book wasn't totally honest, although it was a good start and probably the best I could have done at the time. I thank God I chose to continue growing from there. If I believed in miracles, I would call the effect of that purge of feelings one of the miracles of my life.

Writing *Letters to Mary* hammered home the truth that I was responsible for my own experiences. Somehow it showed me that the chaotic situations and angry people around me represented issues I needed to confront in myself. In essence, my unresolved anger and my unwillingness to forgive were symptoms of the self- hatred that I hadn't released.

The letters described the most painful part of my life—a time so intense that up until quite recently, I felt physical pain each time I re-read those pages. A part of me dreamed of getting rid of *Letters to Mary* and forgetting I had ever written it. In the end, I made the difficult decision to share those pages.

Finally I realized that there must be many other people struggling with the same desperate feelings I had finally expressed in the manuscript. It might be helpful for someone else to see how far down I had to go before I came back up for air. Maybe the message was important; if I got better, anyone can.

I also felt it was valuable to let readers understand that each crossroad

I reached had given me an opportunity for choice. Would I move forward, stand still, regress? The decision was always mine. Writing and keeping *Letters to Mary* was a choice that supported healing. I saw that immediately and it gave me courage to make other choices that were just as positive. My life had never changed because of luck—change occurred because I made a conscious decision to look for another way to exist.

Staying trapped in rage was sure, slow suicide. I know now that this was part of the reason I had made the suicide pact in the first place. I was dying on many levels, and in some ways I was already dead. It had always seemed preferable to me to leave a relationship first, before someone else had a chance to walk out on me. This situation was no different. Why should I wait around for the years of disease to kill me in their own time; I would do it myself.

Writing and keeping *Letters to Mary* finally pushed me over the edge—after I wrote it, life became more appealing. When I looked honestly at who I was, my feelings of guilt, although still strong, became less important. I hoped that the people who might be angry about what I had written would find the courage to tell me, and then we could all clear the air.

Happy Birthday, Linda

Right after I finished the manuscript, I celebrated my 31st birthday, feeling newly born. It was a wonderful experience that few people seemed to understand. Although I was bursting at the seams, I kept the new, tentative feelings of wonder to myself as I turned to face and clear the next set of hurdles.

Letters to Mary was screaming to be seen by eyes other than my own, and I could no longer deny the natural progression of the creative process by refusing to let this happen. But my wonderful sister could not be the first person to see the unfinished manuscript. It had always been hard for us to talk one-on-one about how we felt, and I worried that she might be intimidated by seeing my feelings in print. Just beginning to deal with my own discomfort, I consciously decided to postpone dealing with hers.

I knew that someday I would share the book with Mary, but I didn't know when. The thought of putting my work in the mail terrified me, and calling her and reading out loud it was out of the question. After rereading what I had written to her, I knew how ambivalent I was about Mary's role in my life. To me, she represented change, something I thought I desperately wanted but had always managed to avoid.

So I chose my psychiatrist as the first person to read the book. I handed it to him with a tremendous sense of relief. Much later, I shared it with a few friends and group members. Months after that, I sent Mary a copy. I know she got the book and read it, but we have never discussed it.

When I started looking into publication, I was told that the book wasn't finished—where were the beginning and the end? An agent who read it said she felt suspended in mid-air. I refused to discuss the beginning, and at that point was unable to visualize an end, so I dropped the project. I couldn't imagine telling my psychiatrist—let alone the general public—that *Letters to Mary* was the latest result of a suicide pact that dated back to 1981!

I continued to deal with guilt about exposing myself, my family, and some of what we had been through to the general public. Did I want to do that? Would anyone in my family ever speak to me again? Did I care? There were a number of reasons I felt such ambivalence.

A New View of the World

When I wrote *Letters to Mary,* I was angrier than I had ever been. Making the book public at that time would have done two things:

1) If members of my family read the book (I wasn't sure they would), they might begin to acknowledge my true feelings; and

2) I would finally have found a way to let them know that I blamed them, among others, for my illness. They knew I was angry and must have realized that part of my anger was directed at them, but I had never found a way openly to discuss my feelings.

On the other hand, I was reluctant to share the manuscript because I wanted a guarantee that my family would be around when I needed them. Publishing the manuscript was a risk I wasn't sure I was ready to take.

I was still not dealing honestly with the part of me that enjoyed the excitement of rage. I wrote the manuscript in a "see what the world has done to me" mode, hoping it would make me feel better. But the process of writing showed me how much of my life was my own responsibility. My excitement at finishing the book passed quickly because I realized how much still had to be done.

It was a relief to get the conflicts within me—especially those that involved my family, out in the open. At least four significant changes happened as a direct result of writing *Letters to Mary.* First, I felt safe enough to write again, even if only to someone who lived so far away. Second, I had finally expressed the bottled-up feelings that I had been so reluctant to claim. Third, I had managed to hold on to my work after it was finished. Finally, I found a person to show it to, someone I trusted.

The more subtle changes that occurred were immeasurable. Writing the book also helped me confront the way I was treating my sister. In my mid-twenties, Mary and I had agreed that she was the person I would call on for help if I became too sick to care for myself. We had discussed it calmly and decided that if I became crippled, I would live with her until we figured out what else to do with me. It was a tremendous relief to get that settled, but after we made the agreement, I felt myself developing an unhealthy dependence on her, anticipating an event that had not occurred.

Of course, after I wrote the suicide pact, everything changed.

The pact meant that only one of two things could happen: I would get well or I would kill myself. Either way, I would never be permanently dependent on anyone.

As I began to work this through and see how the pact had changed things, I finally was able to love Mary for herself, not for what I expected from her. With great joy I realized that I finally had a set of principles to guide my life—even if they were the rules of a suicide pact. I could take all my experiences and plans and decide whether they fit into the structure of the pact. My life had become simple.

The process of writing *Letters to Mary* also drastically changed the way I dealt with other people—family members, group members, and my peers at work. I became more honest about expressing my feelings and more verbal in my relationships, learning to ask directly for what I wanted. My negative dependence on others was beginning to turn into more positive requests for support, and I spent less time complaining. The random way I had lived my life was losing its appeal.

As I changed, the people around me also seemed to change their ways of dealing with me. A second set of friends and acquaintances gradually wandered out of my life, and others came rushing in. I began the process of leaving the work for which I was trained to enter a field that simply felt more comfortable. All that movement made me a little anxious, but I knew it was for the best.

Writing *Letters to Mary* was exactly the push I needed to start expressing myself again. After it was finished, I continued to fill all my spare time with writing, sharing every word of it with my psychiatrist. He kept the copies I gave him because I was still fighting wild urges to throw them away. Soon enough, however, I became so obsessed with the desire to write that I even had trouble throwing away grocery lists. At home, I kept the piles of work close beside me until they grew so heavy and high that I began to lose track of how much I had written.

Then a new panic surfaced. I was terrified at the thought of something happening to all that work. I had finally found the courage to write—what if I lost it now? I began to make copies and stash them in odd corners. I had come full circle—from destroying all evidence of my writing to trying to ensure that it would live forever.

Fire, theft, and water damage were always on my mind. I dreamed of winds sweeping through the house and carrying my papers away.

Crying, I would run out the door just in time to see fluffs of white paper floating off in the distance, gone forever. My psychiatrist helped me tremendously during this time. We sat and discussed the probability of various natural catastrophes occurring in Falls Church, Virginia, as if it was a perfectly natural topic of conversation.

I worked slowly through two sets of related feelings: the loss I was beginning to feel after throwing out all my writing for ten years, and the fears stirred up when I finally allowed myself to write uncensored. I mourned for those discarded papers as if my best friend had died. I grieved for the years thrown away, the feelings unacknowledged, and the resulting pain in my body. But during that time, I also began to make up for the lost years, producing volumes of work about topics that had never seemed particularly interesting to me before.

XIII. SPLASH!

Even though I was beginning to tackle many of the issues I needed to deal with, I still felt terrible. I preferred to live in the period between my last two surgeries, comparing every current ache with the way I had felt during that time. At least, now the pain was bearable without massive doses of drugs.

As I took stock of my body—the way I looked and moved after all these months of torturous pain, surgery, and misuse, I felt the need to do something about it. My muscles were atrophying, I was stiff, and I could barely find strength to lift a paper clip.

Earlier in my life—it seemed like centuries earlier—I had joined a spa and gone in for regular workouts. Now just the thought of lifting weights put me through the ceiling. But I remembered the swimming pool at the spa and how good it felt to swim for a few minutes—up until the time my tendon snapped. I couldn't imagine volunteering for any more physical activity than was absolutely necessary, but I knew that I had to start moving my body.

Swimming and walking were the only sports recommended for people with arthritis. My feet hurt too much to do any fast walking, so I decided to reinvestigate swimming. One of my friends at work swam every day, so one day I went with her to check out the locker room and the pool. I wanted to see how many doors I'd have to open, how far I would have to walk, and if I could get in and out of the pool.

All of those calculations were necessary because of the pain. It left me very little energy and made it impossible for me to pull myself out of the water. The pool had a lift for physically handicapped students, but I would have to wait around for someone to get the key every time I wanted to use it. My friend pointed out that getting me into the pool wasn't a problem—it was getting me out that might take some time. She volunteered to boost me out at the end of my swim if I could hold on to the railing as she pushed. I thought about it for a while longer and then decided to take the plunge.

I was still waking up very early each morning to give myself time to get dressed for work. If I planned to swim during lunch, I would have to move fast. I remembered how my sister Mary and I had slept in our school uniforms so we would have enough time to race outside and play tag before the bus came each morning. Getting dressed and undressed took so long and was so painful that I considered wearing my bathing suit to work under my clothes, but decided instead that I would find a way to speed up my movements.

It took much longer for me to walk from the locker room to the pool than I had planned. It even took longer to bend down and get into the water. With so little control over my movements, I thought I'd drown if I jumped in. My first swim measured seven lengths of the pool, using only one stroke. Every time I stopped moving, I thought I'd die. As my friend pushed me out, I was swearing so loudly I'm sure even the deaf people in the pool heard me. One of the things I screamed was that I'd never get back in that pool again. But I had made a commitment to swim three times a week for six months. After six months, if I wanted to, I could stop. I started swimming the first week of January that year and swam three times a week for the next three years.

I swam for the first time (and swore it was my last) on a Monday. Two days later I was back at my friend's desk bugging her to hurry up and get in the pool. The second time in the water, I swam only five lengths. I stayed at five lengths for a month, increased to seven, then added one or two laps a month. I stopped adding laps when I reached a half mile.

Each time I got into the pool, I felt better about myself. I was successfully performing a sport! I went into the locker room with "the girls" every Monday, Wednesday, and Friday, developing a healthy respect for my friends who carried gym bags. And I lost all desire to run down joggers with my car.

As time went on, my body became less my enemy and more my friend. My joints and muscles grew flexible, I built up stamina, and because of the muscles I was developing, I began to put on some weight. But it was slow going, and a full year passed before I noticed any real changes. During that first year, swimming helped ease the pain in my entire body—except my feet. They remained achy, lumpy, and swollen no matter what I did. Now, almost four years into my swimming routine, even my feet feel better. My success in the pool gave me courage to try to succeed at other physical activities. I found that the more I expected of my body, the more it did.

Success Is Not So Bad

The first time I had to miss swimming because of the flu, I panicked, sure that I'd never be able to swim again. I had a fear that if I missed one day in the pool, my joints would freeze and all the benefit I had gained would be lost.

I finally noticed a pattern in these thoughts. It seemed that each time I started something—anything—and allowed myself to enjoy it, I also created mental scenarios of loss and devastation. As I continued to work on the activity, I would slowly began to believe that it was okay for me to succeed, even to have a little fun. But I knew I had to stop torturing myself with thoughts of doom.

I thought that maybe I just needed time to adjust to the fact that I was getting better, but this wasn't the case. It became clear that I had to confront a deeply ingrained belief that someone was waiting to grab me and break my kneecaps every time I allowed myself to feel a little perky. I had become an extremely paranoid person and was living my life based on this paranoia. I realized I suspected "life" of working purposely against me. And for possibly the thousandth time, I found myself asking why getting well was so complicated.

The habits and thought patterns of most chronically ill people take a long time to develop, and they seem to take even longer to throw off. Each time I entered a new level of healing, I had to confront and dismantle a whole new set of fears and beliefs. This paranoia was one of the worst examples.

After four years of swimming on a regular basis, I know the process is working for me. But it took more than time to build trust. I try not be fanatical about anything, but I will go to just about any length to manipulate my schedule so that I can swim. Swimming has become as necessary to me as breathing and eating. It represents freedom and life. Each time I get in the water and start to move, I'm thrilled by doing something I thought would be taken from me forever: controlling the movements of my own body. As I swim, I feel complete awe and appreciation for each part of my body and how perfectly it works.

Locker room conversation is usually dominated by complaints— about the showers, the chlorine in the water, the crowded pool. I couldn't care less. All I need to do is see blue water or smell chlorine and I totally relax. For someone who lived so long as a prisoner of her own body, the movement of swimming is as precious as gold.

XIV. TURNING PAGES

About a month before I started swimming, my sister Mary and her husband were in town for a visit. During that visit, she and I spent a day shopping in Georgetown. Late that afternoon we went to the "Yes" bookstore, known in the Washington area for a good collection of materials on various aspects of self-help and healing. We browsed for a while and found ourselves searching through a pile of books by one author, Catherine Ponder. Mary chose *The Prospering Power of Love,* and I chose *Open Your Mind to Prosperity.* We each agreed to read our own books and swap when we were finished.

Back home, I put the book away and didn't think about it again until two months later. Then one night in February, I found the bookstore bag, containing the Ponder book and two others. The title embarrassed me. How had I managed to buy such a book? Immediately, I realized that my embarrassment and anxiety were telling me something: I needed to read it.

I had always run from anything that made me feel anxious or embarrassed. Now I could use those feelings to identify concepts, people, and situations that I needed to confront. I picked up the book, tired of being embarrassed about my search for better health and a better life. I wanted to shed the constant impulse to hide myself and what I did from other people. I needed to find a way to be proud of who I was, whatever that involved.

Obviously I wanted more prosperity, or I wouldn't have bought the book. Buying it represented the start of my search for a richer, more beautiful life, not just improved physical health. The title and the bright green and gold cover represented a richness I had begun to crave. Still, I couldn't deny that I felt silly— almost like a bad girl—openly wanting and trying to prosper.

Opening the book, I remembered that I had heard the name Catherine Ponder before, and vaguely associated it with the topic of God. If this book was about God, then the words "religion" and "spirituality" could not be far behind. My need to confront my beliefs about religion and spirituality was on my list, but I had successfully ignored those items until that moment. To top it off, here were the words "prosperity" and this woman's name on the same page. I stood there balancing the concepts of God, spirituality, religion, and prosperity, and something told me I was in for the confrontation of my life.

Opening the Book

The first night, I was only able to read the list of other books she had written. Such titles as *Dare to Prosper!*, and *Pray and Grow Rich* set my hair on end, but *The Millionaire From Nazareth* almost put me in a coma. I didn't sleep at all that night.

The next night I tackled the copyright page (Unity School of Christianity!!!) and the Table of Contents. Just reading the blurb about chapter seven made my head spin—it was all about tithing. Somewhere in the back of my mind I knew that tithing meant "giving"—actually giving money away!

The third night I read the introduction. I was totally annoyed because she started out with testimonials. Reading about other people's progress meant nothing to me. Why should I care about people I didn't even know? The stories couldn't possibly be true anyway. Those ridiculous testimonials were a perfect excuse not to read the book. Here I was, trying to avoid comparing myself with anyone, and this woman was urging me to imitate the successes of others.

But I kept reading. It seemed crazy to quit before I even got beyond the introduction, and I knew myself well enough to recognize the symptoms of resistance to progress. I decided to ignore the testimonials and plunge into the book, so on the fourth night I began reading Part I: Basic Methods for Demonstrating Prosperity. That night did help me get my right arm and shoulder into pretty good shape: I spent the next two hours reading one sentence at a time, then throwing the book across the room.

I read the first chapter several times. In it, the author defined poverty as a "sin." She described the feelings of guilt people experience when they want to prosper. She defined prosperity as "health, harmony, peace of mind, and financial plenty," and talked about the bible as a book of wealth. In this first chapter, she also suggested affirmations people might use to open themselves to prosperity.

I saw myself clearly in her words. As I read and re-read the chapter, I felt angry, excited, fascinated, and disgusted all at the same time. I admitted to myself that I had always seen the bible as a book of punishment, guilt, and painful death. I admitted that confusion about what I wanted was my way of hiding from the fact that I craved a better life but didn't know how to find it. I saw that my beliefs were in direct contradiction to what I wanted, and that these conflicting feelings, wants, and beliefs were keeping me from living my life. Something in me said, "This is it. These are the beliefs I need to confront and change." But another voice told me, "Burn the book. Stop searching. This task is bigger than you—you can't do it."

Up Against the Wall

So instead of burning the book, I threw it. Each time a sentence hit a nerve, the book hit the wall. But it wouldn't disappear; the book was always there in the morning after the final evening toss, grinning at me and calling me to finish what I had started.

My fear and anger continued—directed at the message of this book, its author, and the way it seemed to strip me of all my defenses. Simple sentences or paragraphs would touch me in a way that I had never been touched before. All the while I read, I knew the concepts before me were nothing new—they had all been spoken or written many times. But as I pored over each page, I felt like a child just beginning to read. I was discovering a new world—one in which I might have a chance to be happy. I was discovering the world of hope.

Although I've given up trying to intellectualize exactly what was going on in me just before and during this time, I will venture a guess that all the work of the last four years was finally beginning to pay off. It seemed that the purpose of those years was merely to prepare me for the real awakening that began with the purchase of the book.

For a long time, I had been angry with myself for being slow to open my mind—four years seemed like forever. Now I'm much more accepting of the fact that some people take longer than others to deal with the task life presents us with: lovingly accepting responsibility for our own lives. I avoided that responsibility until I found myself drowning in the pain of a crippling disease.

Desire to keep reading soon overrode my feelings of anger. Each time I picked up the book, I understood something that I had previously found confusing, or saw something that I was sure hadn't been on a page the last time I read it. I was consumed with hope. I started copying paragraphs and pages to carry around with me so that when I felt discouraged, they could help me through the storm.

Clean Up, Clear Out

The second chapter of the book stirred up another major conflict. It focused on various ways to clean out my life by getting rid of things I no longer used or wanted. I could start by cleaning out closets, cars—any place that was a haven for clutter. The basic message was: get rid of what you don't want, to make room, literally and figuratively, for what you do want.

That message, so basic and logical, presented a dilemma: Even though I owned many things that I didn't want, I was certain that I would never get what I did want. The idea that I didn't want to be left empty-handed sounded like a hollow rationalization, even to me. Then I reasoned that I was only keeping things I might need later, which was also a lame excuse. If I hadn't used something in seven years, when would I use it?

Overcoming my resistance to the clean-up process, I began to assess my belongings and estimated that I didn't use, wear, or want more than half of the things I owned. On further investigation, I realized that it was much more than that. Giving away everything I really didn't want would leave me with almost nothing.

It wasn't easy to confront the fact that I was unconsciously collecting things—valuable or worthless by dollar amount—that I didn't want or use. I told myself that what the book suggested was an oversimplification at best, and probably pure baloney. But something pushed me to continue, and as I did, I learned something that I would have preferred to keep under wraps. Giving things away didn't appeal to me. I would rather throw them out.

I knew I was mistrustful and a little greedy, but it was depressing to realize how hard it was for me to give. Before reading this book, I had clung to whatever I believed was mine, not caring that someone else might treasure what I found worthless. I struggled with my fear of letting go and my growing desire to learn to give, wondering if my ego could tolerate much more exposure.

Between my bitterness about poor health and the mediocrity of my life, I had become a very self-centered person. Self-centered people don't usually enjoy giving, and I was no exception. For 20 years, I had whined about what fate had withheld from me. There was no room left in my heart for generosity—and I was as stingy with myself as with anyone else.

Then began the phase of giving things away. Friends, charities, family members, no one was exempt from my ill-assorted care packages. Sorting through my things, I became lost in memories. I remembered people giving to me—materially, financially, and otherwise—but had only vague recollections of what I had given in return. When I had given, it had been out of obligation or to get something in return. Giving for the fun of it was new territory.

I continued to move through the pages of the book and through my possessions. The clean-up campaign stirred up so many feelings that I began having nightmares. One night I dreamed that I was in a room full of doors. Behind each one was a pile of rotting bones. It was a perfect dream. What else could I have expected to find?

Learning to Give

Even through the turmoil, I realized that incredible changes were going on inside me. Amazing to think that such a simple process could shake up so much bitterness and resistance! Each time I thought I had nothing left to give, the next week I'd fill two more bags and give them away. Occasionally, I could even give something without immediately wanting it back. I celebrated these times, as though I had aced a major exam. Gradually the process became easier until one day I began to enjoy it. And as I looked around my cleared out, cleaned up living space, I began to feel my mind clearing out as well.

If I could point to one statement in the book that affected me the most, it would be this one from the second chapter: "....remind yourself that the lack of order first exists within you."

Holding off feelings of paranoia, I laughingly told myself that this woman, who appeared to know exactly what was going on in my mind and heart, had been spying on me. As I opened to the ideas in her book, it became my first real working tool for building the kind of life I wanted.

Even though some of the concepts and activities presented in the book bothered me, I decided to follow the exercises to the letter. I was still confused about my negative reactions. Did they indicate a deep-seated resistance to change, or did I truly know what was right for me? I decided to stop asking questions and just get busy. Otherwise, I would never know.

I threw myself completely into the activities, feeling foolish and praying that no one would find out what I was doing. But I was determined to go through with the entire process. Each time I felt like giving up, I reminded myself how well the book described me; it had identified my most serious and basic problems. With each new chapter, I uncovered more and more parts of myself that I wanted to change. I felt scared, but hopeful.

Doing the exercises in the book helped me deal with two major obstacles. It had always been easy for me to identify what I didn't what, but what I wanted had remained unclear. The exercises helped me visualize my desires down to the last detail. Changing focus from negative to positive made me feel much better. No more would I settle for mediocrity. I would no longer use phrases like, "It doesn't matter" or "Someday I'll get used to it," to describe the way my life was going.

Another crucial change occurred as I opened my mind to this author and her ideas. I located a church twenty minutes from my home that based its ministry on metaphysical principles similar to those expressed in the book.

Finding a Community

I read the book a number of times before noticing an address given in a later chapter to help people like me find support. Just before I noticed the address for the first time, I had made a conscious decision to find specific support for what I was trying to do with my life. I didn't intend to join a church, and it came as a big surprise when I realized that was exactly what I was going to do.

I had grown up mistrusting God and religion. As soon as I could, I stopped going to church. The years I did attend—even when I was very young—filled me with fear. I was uncomfortable with what was being taught, and didn't want God to see me nodding agreement to ideas I didn't believe. Afraid to decide what I did believe and even more afraid not to, I felt like a liar and a coward. When the struggle became too intense, I focused on the latest available disaster and left my discomfort about God for another time.

As I thought about joining the new church, I made room in my mind to consider the possibility that I had limited my life by not questioning the religious concepts I had been taught. Not attending church did solve part of the problem; at least I no longer led a double life. But my refusal to deal with God and religion had frozen my spiritual development.

I realized that this was symbolic of the frozen joints and muscles in my body. Because I had refused to deal with issues basic to my survival, my hands barely managed to feed me; my feet barely got me to the toilet in time to empty my bladder. My body, ravaged inside and out, was a symbol of my lack of inner peace and unity. I turned from God out of fear and anger, and ran straight into physical and mental chaos.

Picking up where I had left off years earlier, I allowed myself to consider spirituality and religion as two separate concepts. I saw myself in the little green uniform of my school—sitting, kneeling, and chanting in church—knowing that those countless hours did nothing to enhance my understanding of God. Why was it necessary to belong to and sit in a church to know God?

Along with this awakening came the release of my anger toward the religion in which I had been raised. It dawned on me that there was nothing wrong with my family's religion, it just wasn't right for me. This new way of looking at the situation gave me an incredible sense of freedom. People looked different to me and when I looked in the mirror, I barely recognized myself.

In the middle of the fifth year of my five-year suicide pact, I realized that I had almost missed the boat. In a flash, I knew that all my running to doctors or healers—although crucial in helping me reach this point—had not cured me in the past and would not cure me now. Well into the fifth year, when I had thought I would either be dead or running marathons, I finally understood what I needed to do. I had to confront my beliefs, decide whether I liked them, and find a way to change what I didn't like—without judgement and with forgiveness. I had to decide on a purpose for my life, and then get busy.

My entire life had been spent dancing around the needs and desires of people and organizations that seemed stronger and more important than

I was. I had lived in a way that had literally broken my bones. Now I had begun to believe that there were people who could dance with me and support me as I changed, people who would not try to run my life based on their own needs. I was finding the strength to move forward without asking for approval, and knew that as soon as I figured out who I was and what I believed, I could proudly tell the world.

For five years, I had been isolated in my determination to heal or die. Now I was committed to live in the best way I could. The time had come for me to find a group of people who also wanted to live, and to join with them in spirit. After visiting the church twice, I decided to join. The minister, the people in the congregation, and my commitment to develop a positive connection with this world kept me going, and I began to change the old tapes that had run my mind for thirty-one years.

This non-denominational ministry offered me a group of people who had come through the same struggles I had, and a minister who encouraged us to find out who we were. Looking for, finding, and attending this church showed me that I was almost ready to stand on my own.

As I became actively involved in the church and began to live by the principles I wanted to believe, I felt it was also safe to stop my individual therapy. Around the same time, my rheumatologist decided to move to another state, leaving me in the care of another physician in his practice. I saw the new doctor twice and never went back, and have received no treatments for rheumatoid arthritis since that day. Soon after that, I stopped going for acupuncture treatments; then I quit group therapy.

Discovering Meditation

I had found a comfortable way to live my life. The new principles that I was learning (really as old as mankind) gave me hope, freedom from the past, and a way to forgive myself. But most important of all, my new way of life reintroduced me to the healing qualities of meditation.

During each church service, our minister led us through a period of meditation. Meditation was not new to me. I had tried it in college and given up in despair. Instead of clearing my mind and leaving me peaceful, it left me more frantic and out of control than when I had started. But the type of meditation the minister used was different—it was "led" instead of "free." Her voice leading us through a 15 or 20 minute period, gave me something to hold on to as I practiced releasing the chatter running through my mind. Meditation left me feeling extremely peaceful, knowing more clearly what was right for me. And what was right for me seemed to stray further and further from the norm every day.

Meditating became such a crucial element in my life that I wanted to expand and improve my skills. I quickly found a class and soon I was meditating two or three times a day, feeling better and better by the minute. It took me a long time to trust the intuition I was developing.

What seemed clear to me when I was relaxed and uncluttered became complicated and almost ridiculous when shared with others. I quickly learned to keep quiet about what I was doing until I felt strong enough to deal with criticism. As I became more comfortable with meditation, most people stopped asking me what I was doing. Those who did left my explanations unchallenged.

After meditating for a number of months, I began to take risks and live in ways that I thought would never be possible. It became clear that working full-time at an "okay" job would no longer do. I wanted to work at home, where I would be free to write, meditate, swim, and grow at my own pace. That desire developed into reality more quickly than I ever dreamed it would.

XV. MOVING OUT

Because of the problems I was having with my hands, my employers had temporarily transferred me to the publications unit of the organization. My original teaching job was being cut, but I was offered an opportunity to consider two other jobs within the publications unit. As the time came for me to discuss these jobs with my boss, I realized that I couldn't take either one. To do so would be to risk my health again by working at something that was in direct opposition to my needs. But still I was afraid; my moods swung from excitement to terror.

As my boss began describing the responsibilities of the two jobs, I wasn't sure what I was going to say. All at once, my fear of a life spent fighting illness overcame my fear of change, and I told her that I wasn't interested in either one. She was surprised, saying that the meeting was not going as she had planned. I was shocked at the fact that I had gotten the words out of my mouth.

Fear was still running the show, although it should have been clear that I had been preparing to do this for four years. Whatever my motivation, I had finally done the right thing for myself at the right time. It may sound like a paradox, but leaving full-time, permanent employment to seek a new and better life was a first step. I had finally begun to take care of myself and ensure my own success. Two months after that conversation with my boss, I began to work as a free-lance writer. Opportunities came to me as if out of nowhere and my life flowed as it had never done before.

During that time, I also found a way to allow myself the freedom and luxury of living alone. Being by myself was no longer one of my many fears. So many of my dreams had come true! I felt better than I had in years; I had my own home and was working there; my relationships had improved tremendously; I was on my way to forgiving myself and others; I wanted to live. But one fantasy I had when I started the suicide pact hadn't become reality.

Five years had not been enough time to get my life in order, indeed, it had just begun. It seemed that the more happiness I found, the more I wanted. So at the end of the original five years, I gave myself two more. My five-year suicide pact had become a seven-year plan.

Learning to Love

In the sixth year of my pact, I met the man who is now my husband. But before I allowed myself the commitment of marriage, I first had to deal with my reluctance to commit totally to my own life. In the months before our wedding, I released the option of suicide completely. My vows included a promise to both of us that I would stick around. Because of our commitment to loving ourselves, Richard and I are able to give each other the kind of love and support that was once only a fantasy.

In the final months of the seventh year, I find myself becoming my own parent—dealing with the world of health and learning how to live to the fullest. I continue to write and have developed an adult education course based on perceiving life in a positive way. The course fulfills my need to teach in a less judgmental manner. Neither attendance nor grades are mandatory. Each of my students makes his or her own way through the concepts I offer, and the constant need to repeat the things I have learned helps reinforce my own convictions about the things I most need to know.

I attended church regularly for about two years, and then decided to join a weekly support group.* These days, on my occasional visits to church, I feel a tremendous amount of love. I also attend yearly workshops given by Arnold and Selma Patent as a way of expanding my support group experiences. The love and support I get from my group is the most I could desire. We meet to support each other, to honor God, and to acknowledge his presence within us as purpose, talent, and creativity. Because of my commitment to this experience, each week my connection to and understanding of God expands, along with my joy at being alive.

In the past, no matter what I did, I felt like a failure. It meant nothing that by most standards my accomplishments were significant. These seven years have helped make it clear that it is not what I do but how I feel that ensures my happiness. When I feel peaceful, everything I do feels like success, from scrubbing the floor to writing a book. When I feel anxious or angry, no matter how much I accomplish, it feels like failure. The members of my support group help me keep this life-saving revelation in focus.

Because I am more trusting than I used to be, my movement toward inner peace no longer consists of jumping from one self- improvement program to the next. Although I am aware of the different ways of approaching the principles I am beginning to live, I intend to stay on one path until it no longer feels comfortable to do so.

My love for my immediate family continues to grow. My eyes have opened to the fact that, at some level, every family deals with mental and physical illness and that we were not, are not, alone in our struggles. I have begun to see my family and the families around me as people who help me grow and learn the lessons of life, and I'm beginning to feel the truth of the idea that all of us on this earth are part of the same family.

I am still working on becoming my own authority, releasing the need to blame. It's taken some time for me to make peace with the medical profession. Now when I need to see a doctor, I stay actively involved. I ask questions, take time to consider any recommended treatments, and say no when I feel that a treatment is unnecessary or not in my best interests. I also practice self-forgiveness for the judgments I have made and the anger I have felt toward an entire profession.

Releasing Consequences

Three of the consequences of my long illness are anemia, a dry left cornea, and a periodic need for physical chaos. My body does not tolerate iron supplements, so I deal with the anemia through an iron-rich diet and multiple vitamins. A nearby university medical center monitors the chronic dryness in my eyes, and has also gotten me involved in a research study. I had an interesting problem with my cornea, but it is healing slowly, with the unexpected bonus of significantly improved vision. I now recognize the warning signals of impending physical crisis and can often stop it before it happens. When for some reason I don't, and chaos strikes, I do my best to love myself during the recuperation period and to get back into the cycle of physical peace. As I learn from these situations, my physical and mental health continue to improve.

A recent blood test for RA indicators showed that certain blood levels remain "higher than they should be." Because of this, I have been encouraged by a physician to again take medication for arthritis. I have chosen not to, for a number of reasons.

I find it difficult to even consider comparing my 34-year-old body, that until recently experienced one disease after another, to a chart of "healthy" norms. In my opinion, spending time worrying about getting things "back to normal" would only lead to disaster, probably in the form of another stress-related illness. After what I've been through, the concept of "normal" has lost its meaning.

Five years ago, thoughts of what might happen to my body 20 years from now could send me running to the doctor's office. Now I'm no longer scared by discussions of what might happen to me when I'm 50 or 60. I will continue to trust my own feelings of peace and physical comfort, especially when doing otherwise means returning to a cycle that offered me so little help. It's not that I never go to the doctor—I do. I have yearly checkups in the necessary areas, and if I happen to fall in the tub, I take the pain medication they give me in the emergency room.

The two reasons for my dependence on doctors and medication—pain and fear—rarely haunt me any more. When they do, they are usually not severe enough to lead me back to taking medicines that compound my problems. It is my choice to trust that as I continue to grow in self-love and forgiveness, the process of releasing rheumatoid arthritis will also continue. I make this choice and accept full responsibility for it.

I still meditate as a way of maintaining the peacefulness I need to find direction, creativity, and continued growth. Like swimming, meditation is not an end result, but a means to an end. It is part of the inner work that keeps the outer part of my life knowing and peaceful.

I would like to describe all the wonderful things I believe will happen in the days to come, but one of my resolutions is to live in the moment I have. And although tomorrow still concerns me, I am much more capable of living in now. I will say one thing about the future: my participation in it will be a process requiring commitment and recommitment for each day that I am alive. And as I continue to release the two illusions of fear and pain, that commitment becomes one of joy.

QUESTIONS, ANSWERS, INFORMATION

I'm ending this book with three categories of information. The first section consists of answers to the questions I'm most frequently asked. Some of the questions are specific to me and my past and current health; others are about the healing process in general. Although I can't solve other people's problems, I do feel I know where they might start looking to find answers for themselves.

The second section is general advice. People often ask me for tips as they begin the process of fighting an illness or changing patterns. This section is based on the assumption that the reader is fully aware of the changes that need to be made. I also assume a willingness to take responsibility for initiating the healing process. I approached this section remembering that I started the process of healing with two major complications: guilt and fear. The suggestions are geared toward people who are not ready to go on the Phil Donahue Show just yet.

The third section is a list of books, tapes, and programs I have read, listened to, and followed, that have helped me in my healing process.

Appendix I
Personal Questions

Are you completely free of pain?

No, but I intend to be. Each time I meditate and follow intuition instead of logic, I feel better. I see becoming pain-free as a process that grows in me as I let go of guilt and fear. I have less pain today than I had six months ago. And I intend to be in even less pain six months from now.

This question brings up an interesting point. There are days when I notice I'm limping—something I used to do constantly. On those days, I ask myself why—am I really in pain? Usually, the answer is no. Limping is something I tend to do when I'm feeling mental pain, don't want to do something I feel I must do, or when I am working toward another major change. For me, any kind of pain represents resistance. I describe this phenomenon because I want to emphasize that for me, pain is two dimensional: physical and mental. One kind of pain has never existed for me without the other. Each time I have tried to separate the two, I have caused myself incredible anguish.

If you could name one thing you did that helped you the most, what would it be?

Deciding that I wanted to heal. I'm not talking about my conscious mind deciding to heal—of course, on a surface level, I always wanted to feel better. But part of me was working in direct opposition to healing; part of me was willing to live in pain and chaos because they were comfortable and familiar. I didn't want to give up my anger. I'm talking about wanting to heal on a subconscious level, because that is the part of me that seems to have the most power. If I had never honestly decided that I wanted to heal, I never would have.

Do you really feel that coming to terms with God and your spirituality were crucial to your healing?

Yes. I believe that it is my purpose on this earth to know who I am in terms of God and spirituality, and to decide where and how to express my faith. I now enjoy being aware that I believe in God, and developing my spirituality. I also know that if I don't, one of two things will happen.

One, other people will decide for me what I believe. Two, I will wander aimlessly through life believing only in luck. And for me, luck was always bad.

I have suffered both these consequences and I don't intend to deal with either of them again. The only way I can guarantee this is by knowing who I am and what I believe.

I'm not saying that I'm closed to other points of view or that I won't change a belief if I find it no longer works for me. I am saying that I intend to know myself and where I fit in on this earth. For me, developing my spiritual beliefs is the key to success. Everything else is an offshoot of that process.

How do you know where you fit in and what is best for you?

Through intuition gained through meditation. When I started meditating, all I knew was that it helped me feel calm and relaxed, at least for short periods of time. As I continued, the physical relaxation seemed to expand, and I noticed something else happening, too. Answers to the questions that had confused me for years became clear, although I didn't trust those answers or follow through on what I knew for a long time. I didn't realize it at the beginning, but I was developing my intuition through meditation.

When I don't take time to meditate, two things begin to happen almost immediately. First, I become intensely uncomfortable physically. Second, I become confused and return to my past state of not knowing what to do and trying to force things to happen that shouldn't be happening. The result is chaos. Meditating is one habit I don't see myself releasing any time soon.

Have you found a way to be cheerful and happy all the time? Don't you get tired of always needing to grow?

No and sometimes. I constantly deal with the part of me that had free reign for 27 years; the part that was determined to be sick, unhappy, and undeserving. I have managed to lessen the amount of time that I feel unhappy and desperate, and I will continue to move toward feeling happy for as much of my time as I possibly can.

There are days when I say I've had enough of this growth business; that I'm going to do everything I can to make myself miserable. Once I used to say that seriously, now I say it as a way to laugh at myself when I get bogged down. I realize that if I let myself stagnate as I have in the past, I get sick.

I no longer see growing as a choice. I see it as a necessity, for as long as I want to stay physically intact.

Does everyone have to do what you did to get well? It seems like so much trouble.

No, other people don't have to do what I did to get well. They do have to determine what healing or changing means for them, and then follow through with whatever they decide must be done. For some, change will be easier. For others, the path will seem, as mine often did, like torture. For these people, suicide may sometimes seem more appealing than doing what they have to do to heal.

Keep in mind that by the time I decided to change, I had spent 27 years living every facet of my life in a self-destructive manner. Every step I took, literally and figuratively, was sheer torture. Changing meant learning how to think in a new way that would support me and make me feel wonderful, and to stop reinforcing my belief in illness. It took me a while to get the hang of being happy, and there are times when it is still uncomfortable.

Many people I know are at least as old as I was when they begin to desire change. When I look at my life and the ways I have changed, I know that it can be done. It is a matter of asking the questions, "Am I honestly satisfied with the way my life is progressing?" and "What kind of life do I want?"

So where do I start?

That's a tough question for me because I started at the end. I wouldn't exactly recommend a suicide pact as a way to begin the healing process, but again, many people seem to need to hit rock bottom before they decide to change.

If you think you need to change, I would recommend that you look at what is going on in your life and decide whether you like what you see. If not, then be very specific about what you want to change. Many people need help with this step, as I did. For years, I walked around feeling vaguely distressed, depressed, and sick, until it was almost too late.

Therapy and self-help books and programs are excellent ways to start the process. Some solutions present themselves quickly, as did my need to divorce. But it's important to understand that surface solutions are only valuable if they help uncover the real issues. If the basic problems are not addressed and unresolved, they are sure to resurface again and again, in other situations, with other people.

I have friends whose second marriages fail, or who leave jobs they dislike only to find themselves facing again the same problems they thought they had left behind. This is because unresolved problems don't go away. They get worse.

After you act on surface solutions, the real work begins. Look for ways to continue exploring change: acupuncture, therapy, meditation, self-help programs, positive support groups, whatever. The process and the choice of paths is very personal. Contrary to popular belief, once you have decided to change, it can happen quickly.

How long will it take me to change?

First of all, it depends on how long it takes to decide honestly to change. Remember, the conscious and subconscious minds can be roughly described as two different entities, often working against each other. It also depends on where you are in terms of your ability to accept responsibility for growth. In other words, it depends on how much resistance you decide to put in your own way. Blaming, guilt, and refusing to start the process of forgiving are all great ways to resist growth.

Even when people are doing the best they can to grow and change, the process of healing won't be hurried. Each of us has an internal time clock that needs to be honored. As you might have noticed while reading this book, I was constantly annoyed about the length of time it took me to change. I complained about it every chance I got, and sometimes still do. Finally, the psychiatrist I worked with explained the concept of time and healing this way:

If I am preparing a certain recipe, I can gather, chop up, and otherwise prepare the ingredients I need very quickly. But each recipe requires that the ingredients be put together in a certain way and cooked for a specific amount of time. The cake just isn't going to come out right if the ingredients are not mixed properly, or baked for the correct length of time.

There is a similar process for growth, change, and healing. We can do some things, such as prepare ourselves for healing by opening ourselves to the process. But trying to force the process only impedes it.

Some people wonder why they have trouble maintaining intimate relationships when they have not started the process of forgiveness. I was very upset about my own intimate relationships until I realized that I had not developed the qualities in myself that I wanted my partner to have. I thought I had done everything I needed to do to experience a wonderful relationship, when in reality, I hadn't.

My psychiatrist ended his parable there, but I can continue the comparison in answering some other questions:

Does this mean that if you burn the cake you can't ever attempt to make it again?

No. But you would have to spend time and energy running around to gather the ingredients and repeat the process.

Does it mean that you can't play with the recipe to bake the cake more quickly or slowly?

No. But you probably don't know how the cake was supposed to taste. If you want to experience it as it was intended, you must combine the correct ingredients and bake it for the recommended length of time.

How do you know when you are hurrying or delaying the cooking process?

There are a few obvious ways to know this. One way is to realize that you've tried the same recipe 10 times, thinking that you followed it to the letter, but it has never come out right. It's like being in therapy for a long period of time and still feeling pretty sure from the way things are going that you haven't made any progress. We all know people who marry or change jobs frequently with the same discomforting results each time. These people are obviously repeating a pattern.

Should the people involved feel bad about themselves because of this?

No, but they might want to find a way to be more honest with themselves and the people around them. I was able to do this through meditating and responding to the insights that came to me.

How much time will it take for me to change?

Time is an interesting concept—it plays an important role for people who want to compare themselves with others. When I was in the stage of constantly complaining about time, I usually got one of two reactions: 1) "You started your healing process at age 27. I'm 47 and still haven't managed to start. Stop complaining." or 2) "Yes, it sure took you a long time. What were you doing in your early 20s when I was busy growing up?"

One woman, a former boss, compares my process to the mid-life crisis many people go through in their late thirties or early forties. We decided that either I'm way ahead of myself or that I've lived so many lousy lives in the past that I just got tired of being miserable! Time is another element that depends solely on point of view, and in the end is totally meaningless. Decide to move forward and you will, at your own pace.

Maybe I was meant to be exactly as I am. What if I was put on this earth to suffer through the exact problems I am trying to change?

I believe that I am drawn to the kinds of situations I experience because of my need to grow in those areas, not because God is trying to punish me. I don't believe that anyone was meant to suffer or be unhappy; I believe people bring suffering on themselves when they refuse to grow or change in the ways they can, or when they accept as reality the destructive thoughts that run through their minds. Before age 27, I had stopped growing in every area, literally making myself miserable. I accepted a totally negative view of reality and lived a life that reflected that belief.

I now believe that God, or the Higher Energy I believe in, wants me to be happy. I believe that even after people go through tremendous life changes, forced or self-initiated, if they continue to believe that they were meant to suffer, they will. If they can go through the same growth process and come out of it believing that they deserve to be happy, they will find a way to become so. I have seen both things happen.

I also believe that it was irresponsibly passive of me to accept circumstances that I didn't like or want in my life. (I am not talking about loving myself as I was. That is a separate issue.) The natural consequences of that irresponsibility were one illness after another, lousy relationships, and a suicidal attitude toward life. When I committed to changing my life to meet my intuitive standards, I began to experience health, the healing of old relationships and the blossoming of new ones, and a positive attitude about my presence on this earth.

What else would you like to try?

There are a few things I'd like to investigate. One is herbal medicine; another is dream work. In addition, I'd like to spend more time experiencing inner peace through meditation and working with my support group. Something tells me that I'll always have a mental list of things I want to try.

If You Have RA...

...and want to get off medication, don't do it until you are ready. If you have a lot of questions about whether you are ready, you aren't.

...and want to see the doctor less frequently, or not at all, don't stop going until you are ready. Again, you will know when the time is right.

...and want to investigate the alternatives, do so slowly and with intention. Scattering your time will only scatter your energy.

...and want to try every alternative because you are afraid not to, please try to focus on one plan at a time. Again, scattering time scatters energy.

...and want to change your job, marital status, or living situation because you think a change will help you feel better, try to stay where you are (unless the situation is abusive) until you are sure you are making a positive move. Jumping from one bad situation to another only encourages feelings of hopelessness.

...and want to get well, know that the process will require you to feel, think, and act in ways that are different from what you do now. This is not a judgement, but a conclusion drawn from working with myself and others who are ill.

...and want to get well, know that you have my support and the support of many other people who are dealing with change. We are with you, and we send you our love.

Appendix II
General Advice

1. Love your neighbors, but don't listen to them.

One thing I learned to do when I began the healing process was to ignore other people's opinions and feelings about everything— doctors, family, friends, the media, everybody. Sad to say, but because I had no self-esteem, up until then the feelings and opinions of other people had meant more to me than my own. People were always telling me that I could not get well—that I should resign myself to having RA for the rest of my life. Although I pretended that what they were saying didn't bother me, it did.

At one time, I stopped seeing nearly everyone I knew because their presence made my task even harder. If the topic became too negative for me to handle, I would leave the room. I almost always ate lunch alone, and meditated during my free time. Until I developed the mental strength to block out negative messages, I was strictly protective of myself. I cancelled my newspaper subscription, and quit watching TV. A few years later, when I decided to reenter the world of the media and other people's opinions, it seemed that there was much less negativity to deal with.

If you are trying to find a way to heal or change, please protect yourself. Stay away from the people and situations that drain the energy you need to progress. There are worse things in life than spending time alone; being with people who reinforce despair and depression is one of them. After a while, these people will either drop out of your life or change with you. Protecting yourself is one way of letting people know that even though you love them, you intend to keep moving ahead.

2. Keep quiet about the changes you are making.

To most people, change is frightening. People tend to resist changing themselves and to feel uncomfortable when they see changes in others. We all have bad habits we want to change, but it's a lot easier to say things like, "You can't teach an old dog new tricks," or "I've tried to change and I can't."

Loudly broadcasting your determination to be happy, thin, rich, or healthy brings up too many questions in people's minds— questions they might not feel comfortable dealing with. Don't let people use you as a way to voice their own anxieties. When the results of your work begins to show, other people who want to change will be able to use you as a role model. It's much more fun that way.

You probably understand that people will know something is going on when you start to change. My fantasy was that I could change my life completely without anyone noticing. Some people will confront you with questions and advice about what's happening. Others will make subtle comments about the differences they see in the way you are acting. Plan to deal with these approaches before the changes begin to show. You can respond to questions, challenges, and comments if you wish, but I don't recommend it unless you feel very secure about what you are doing. I wasn't the least bit secure about changing until I was well into the process. I hope things will be different for you.

In the face of confrontation, I found that saying, "Yes, I'm making some changes but I don't feel comfortable talking about them yet," was an acceptable response. People would either leave me alone or tell me they wanted to hear about what I was doing, whenever I was ready to talk. When I answered defensively, the situation tended to degenerate quickly. Keep yourself out of situations where you have to defend yourself. They only waste precious energy.

3. No matter what part of the process you're in, love yourself.

This is more easily said than done. As a matter of fact, I've got a lot of nerve even writing it down. I was so busy focusing on my surface problems (disease, money, etc.) that the fact that I intensely disliked myself totally slipped my attention.

Anyway, if you are in the shape I was in when I started this process, you can be sure that lack of self-esteem is a problem. If you have trouble believing this, I strongly suggest that you assume it's true and begin to deal with it now. You'll save yourself a lot of time because you won't have to back-track. Trust me on this one.

I recommend that you buy and read a book on self-esteem. One good one is *You Can Heal Your Life,* by Louise Hay. I couldn't figure out what was holding me back in certain areas until I bought her book and tried the mirror exercise. Just one attempt to look in the mirror and tell myself that I loved, approved, and accepted myself showed me exactly what I had to do next. With the help of this book and my support group, I have been working steadily on loving myself just as I am. It would have been a lot easier if I had started the process of building self-esteem when I was 27, but I guess my inner timer just wasn't ready.

If you don't truly love yourself, you won't feel that you deserve to heal. If you don't feel that you deserve to heal, you won't. Learning to love yourself for the changing human being you are is the true beginning of healing.

4. Know that by honestly deciding to change, you will.

Many people truly believe they cannot change. My own feelings of hopelessness and despair revolved around this belief. After I began to believe that change was possible, I found another obstacle in my way: the belief that change could only come slowly and with agonizing effort. Now I recognize that both of those beliefs were untrue.

This is not to say that I never feel stuck, or afraid that I've taken on too much. What has changed is my ability to deal with and release the negative thoughts that still arise. When I feel down, I review the last few years and am amazed at all the changes I've made. This helps keep me going when I feel the need to measure my progress.

If you don't feel you have any major life accomplishments to praise yourself for, look to any success you can remember—no matter how small you think it is—and revel in it instead of wallowing in feelings of hopelessness. Lots of people think nothing good has ever happened in their lives, but if you keep looking, you can always find something positive. Focusing on what has gone well in the past gives you energy to move forward. And some day you will realize that you've changed much more than you ever thought possible.

Some people say that in spite of trying to focus on their successes, they can't seem to shut down the negative voices. It was that way for me in the beginning and I know how frustrating it is. The next section of this book lists a number of books and tapes written by people who have developed excellent strategies to deal with this problem. Please look for some of them, and read them.

After every down period, commit yourself again to change. During every up period, commit yourself to feeling even better.

5. If there are many things about yourself that you want to change, find a way to get started.

After I made it through the ups and downs of deciding whether or not I really wanted to change, I was struck by the overwhelming feeling that I had to change thousands of things about myself, immediately. Because of this feeling, I started my original list of things to try. And because I couldn't identify which part of me needed to change first, I focused on methods of change and let them pave the way. As time went on and I began to know what was important, I was able to work from my own desires, not from a randomly constructed list. But the point is that finding a place to start was the beginning of the process.

It's very easy to say that there's too much to do, and therefore never get started. I know from experience that choosing one thing—anything—and pursuing it leads either to the issue that should be dealt with first, or to the next thing that needs to be confronted. If you can't find a logical way to proceed, write ten things that you want to change on ten slips of paper, drop them in a hat, pick one, and get busy. You'll be amazed at how quickly things happen after that first step.

6. Know that all through the process, you must work on forgiving and releasing everyone, especially yourself.

Forgiving and releasing are ways to let go of the past. The past is over and done; all anyone has is the present moment and hope for the future. Dragging the past into the present or projecting it into the future guarantees that you will stay angry, sad, and resentful. You find yourself living for a time that seemed better, or being bogged down in an experience that you believe has ruined your life.

Many people have problems with the concept of release. They tell me they can't forgive, because the person or organization in question has said or done so many unforgivable things. In truth, they have no intention of forgiving: They want to hold a grudge and refuse to accept any responsibility for the problem. From my experience, it takes two people to start a problem and two people to keep it going, but only one person to lay it to rest.

People who are unwilling to forgive or to accept responsibility aren't "bad" or "wrong." They are, however, setting up consequences for themselves that will not change until they do.

Other people ask me how they can be sure they've forgiven; they think they have but they're not positive. If you aren't quite sure you've forgiven, chances are you haven't.

I have had to forgive, forgive, and forgive some more. Each time I forgave another person, I forgave myself. As the past began to lose its appeal, I moved more fully into the present.

7. What was right for me or for someone else might not be right for you.

You may run into well-meaning people who tell you they have exactly the right answers for you, and that you must follow this advice to the letter. Run, don't walk, from these people. You can be sure that no one else can possibly know what is right for you. Sometimes it's helpful to listen to suggestions, but don't let anyone try to direct your path.

I used to enjoy depending on others. Then if something went wrong, I had someone else to blame. But blaming was a dead end that always left me back where I started. After a while, I developed the confidence to make my own mistakes and take credit for my own successes.

Look at it this way: We had the power to get ourselves into these situations; used constructively, that same power can get us out. Again, my way of knowing what is right for me is through the intuition I gain through meditating. Since I have learned to rely on my own intuition, no one can lead me very far in the wrong direction. And more importantly, I'm no longer stuck with a life that doesn't work.

8. Center your commitment to change on yourself.

I spent a lot of time worrying about other people and their problems before I realized that I had no business worrying about anyone but myself. My life became so simple after this realization— almost too simple for me to handle.

My need to interfere represented my reluctance to confront my own problems. If you find yourself buying self-help books or saving newspaper clippings to give to friends, or in any way trying to run someone else's life, take an honest look at what you're doing. You might find that the person who needs to read those books or articles or take that course is you.

Again, many people react negatively to this advice. I just know that if I had done even half of the things I tried to get other people to do, I would have saved myself a lot of time. After I began taking care of my own problems, I realized that what other people did or didn't do wasn't important. You might find the same thing.

Appendix III
Resources

There are many people who have taken hold of their lives and made important changes. And, some have found a way to share their strategies for change by writing books or making tapes. Allow yourself to reap the benefit of these people's journeys by using their materials, especially if you have haven't been able to change on your own or feel trapped in a life that isn't working.

I know from experience that when we are depressed, even the simple act of buying a book or a tape can seem like too much to handle. And the next step—using what we have purchased—can be even more overwhelming. I also know that the process of change never ends, but to continue, it must begin.

At the beginning of my search, I was confused by the many available programs. I tried to do everything at once, which only added to my anxiety. My solution was to do, read, or listen to only what felt positive, not what I thought I "had to do" or "should be doing." I suggest that you do the same.

I also found it helpful to read some of the books I used into a recorder and listen to them during my free time. Hearing my own voice speaking the positive thoughts of these authors compelled me to keep going when I was ready to give up. As I continued to tape and listen, I began to understand and live by the principles these people had so lovingly shared with me.

I read about or tried many other books and programs in addition to those named below, but they didn't suit my needs as well as the ones I've listed. This list is far from complete; it is simply a catalog of what I liked. Other people may present these same concepts in a way that speaks louder to you. The materials that I spent the most time with are reviewed.

To all the authors, presenters, and people who have helped me, I want to thank you for giving me a piece of your pie. With your help, my first one is whole—and I'm working on my second filling.

BOOKS

You Can Have It All, Death, Taxes, and Other Illusions, Arnold Patent
The author of these books expresses a belief system that I am moving toward accepting. He presents universal principles in a simple manner and includes excellent strategies for change. The support group I attend operates by the guidelines outlined by Mr. Patent.

Love Is Letting Go of Fear, Gerald Jampolsky
This book attracted me later in my healing process. I had made progress in releasing the past but still felt uncomfortable. This book helped me realize what the discomfort was about: my fear of the future. Reading it continues to help me let go of both the past and future so I can live now.

Love Your Disease-It's Keeping You Healthy, John Harrison
I read this book simply because I found the title so amazing. The author lovingly confronts the reader about responsibility and understanding the purpose of illness. I recommend it highly.

Open Your Mind To Prosperity, The Dynamic Laws of Healing, The Healing Secrets of the Ages, Catherine Ponder
These were the first books I read on healing and change. Although I had a hard time dealing with the first one, they were a wonderful way to start.

Spiritual Economics, Eric Butterworth
I spent a lot of time with this book; it was the first one I taped. Reading and listening to it gave me courage.

Higher Creativity—Liberating the Unconscious for Breakthrough Insights, Willis Harman and Howard Rheingold
At first this book frightened me—I started it and put it down many times. I did the affirmations in the back of the book for six months and read every bit of it as slowly as I needed to. I unsuccessfully tried to do the exercises given in the book, but later found myself completing them during meditations or dreams.

Right Brain Experience, Marilyn Zdenek
I went through this book and its program during a vacation. It was a very intense experience that helped me get in touch with the fact that I was barely using the right side of my brain. Two weeks after finishing the program I was able to visualize on the right side of my mental screen during meditations.

Money-love, Jerry Giles
The process of buying this book and reading it left me with one feeling: embarrassment. As I bought it, I kept looking over my shoulder to make sure no one noticed the title. My feelings and behavior only emphasized my need to deal with the issue of money. The book helped me confront many negative thoughts I carried with me about money, its use, and its real purposes. It further helped me understand that I was owned by money and possessions, and helped me continue the process of turning those beliefs around.

You Can Heal Your Life, Louise Hay
This book helped me incredibly with self-esteem, making it clear that after all my work, I didn't have any. I worked with the ideas in this book two hours a day for almost two months. I still refer to the list of possible causes and affirmations in the back of the book.

The Lazy Man's Guide to Enlightenment, Thaddes Golas
This book is great bathroom reading, and I don't say this in jest. Before I got my body working right, I spent a lot of time in the bathroom. It was just what I needed: I could read a concept the way Mr. Golas presented it and then get back to work. As Mr. Golas himself says, "Enlightenment doesn't care how you get there."

Super Learning, Sheila Ostrander & Lynn Schroeder
This book put me touch with the Lozanov Learning Institute, which in turn helped me find an excellent way to reduce studying time. By "accident," I also found the method of studying described an excellent way to do my affirmations.

The Edgar Cayce Collection, Hugh Lynn Cayce, editor
This book increased my interest in dreams, giving me a clearer understanding of how to interpret them. I had always experienced vivid dreams but never gave them much thought until I read this book.

Unlimited Power, Anthony Robbins
Mr. Robbins offers wonderful strategies for clearing the mind of chatter and negative illusions. It should be read in pieces because of the amount of information included.

Taking the Path of Zen, Robert Aithen
Mr. Aithen guides his readers through the art of breathing.

Kindness, Clarity and Insight, Tenzin Gyatso
The concept of karma is simply described by the fourteenth Dalai Lama.

Lupus Novice: Toward Self-Healing, Laura Chester

Do What You Love: The Money Will Follow, Marsha Sinetar

Prosperity's Ten Commandments, Georgiana Tree West

Why Did This Happen to Me?, Joseph Murphy

Body Learning: An Introduction to the Alexander Technique, Michael Gelb

The Revolutionary Way to Use Your Body For Total Energy—The Alexander Technique, Sarah Barker

Focus on Crystals. Edmund Harold

The Crystal Sourcebook: From Science to Metaphysics, John Milewski & Virginia Harford

Autobiography of a Yogi, Paramahansa Yogananda

Mind as Healer, Mind as Slayer, Kenneth R. Pelletier

Holy Bible, Red Letter Edition, Old and New Testaments

The Screwtape Letters, Mere Christianity, C. S. Lewis

Getting Well Again, O. Carl Simonton, Stephanie Matthews-Simonton, James L. Creighton

Super Immunity, Paul Pearsall

Love, Medicine, and Miracles, Bernie Siegel

People of the Lie, The Road Less Traveled, M. Scott Peck

The Wounded Woman: Healing the Father-Daughter Relationship, Linda Schierse Leonard

Anatomy of an Illness, Norman Cousins

The Nature of Personal Reality, The Education of Oversoul Seven, The Further Education of Oversoul Seven, Jane Roberts

Tales for Jung Folk, Richard Roberts

Feeling Good—The New Mood Therapy, David M. Burns

When Bad Things Happen to Good People, When All You've Ever Wanted Isn't Enough, Harold S. Kushner

Health and Healing, Andrew Weil

The Macrobiotic Way, Michio Kushi

Fit for Life, Harvey and Marilyn Diamond

MAGAZINES

"New Realities," Heldref Publications
4000 Albermarle Street
Washington, DC 20016

TAPES

Jon Shore, Light Unlimited Publications
HC 02 Box 943
Cave Creek, Arizona 85331

Lozanov Learning Institute
8719 Colesville Road, Suite 300
Silver Spring, Maryland 20910

Superlearning Inc.
Suite 500
450 Seventh Avenue
New York, New York 10123

Arnold Patent, Celebration of Abundance
Goodkind of Sound
Route 3, Box 365 AA
Sylva, North Carolina 28779
PO Box 336
Piermont, NY 10968

William F. Schwartz, Mind Power Institute
5817 Bywood Drive
Indianapolis, Indiana 46220

Linda Frazer Fleming, PO Box 3175
Falls Church, Virginia 22043

Louise Hay, Hay House
3029 Wilshire Blvd.
Santa Monica, California 90404

Thomas Budzynski, Bio-Feedback Systems
2736 47th Street
Boulder, Colorado 80301
or
Nightingale-Conant Tapes

Dick Sutphen, Master of Life
Box 38
Malibu, California 90265

Inner Guidance Systems
Gwynedd Plaza II, Suite 301
Springhouse, Pennsylvania 19477

Synton Research Inc.
Mail Order Department
175 Fifth Avenue
New York, New York 10010

Alex Jones & Douglas Cutler
Eric Butterworth, Unity, New York
Self-made affirmation tapes

Appendix IV
LETTERS TO MARY

A Sister in Me

Finally
I allowed
the thought
of someone
in

and was surprised
to find you
already there.

Then I looked
in the mirror
as I combed my hair,
stepping into my shoes
I could feel
you there

a slight streak
of you
inside me

A gesture of the hand
a roll of the eye
I remind me
of you
and I didn't even try.

How can anyone
be in me
without my consent?
especially you,
thousands of miles away?

I didn't know
you'd be with me
wherever I go.

I've opened
to the thought
of you
in me

and found a place
I thought
impossible
to be:
the center of me.

August 11, 1985

Dear Mary,

In the past two and a half months, I've started this book three different times, and thrown each one out. Every time I started, I'd get halfway through and throw down my pen and paper. Each time I did that, I'd move to the next stack of paper and pens and write poems. After I finished each poem, I'd type it, making a copy for you. I never sent them.

This day has been hard. I started my book again, but stopped. How can I write to the world at large about things so personal and difficult? I know I have a message to give, yet I need someone I know has the ability to listen and feel what I write. Someone who is able to cry at the sad parts and understand the rage, and who can giggle with me at the humor I've found in dealing with life and rheumatoid arthritis.

That person is you. The person I can trust with my feelings is you. Whatever heartache or joy I earn from writing this book, I'll know I had one person to understand. Thanks for being with me.

I love you,
Linda

Reader Beware

Reader beware
you may not care
for the things
you read
in me.

I've seen the look
of shock
as I unlock
Let others read
my first book
of honesty.

Pressure is there
in the stare
"Close the book
never
open it again
it's not
for my eyes."

They say,
"Everything you say
has been said
before.
Stop this nonsense!
The words
are not yours
to use
and never were."

All that's coming
from them now
is anger
wanting
easy lies.

I give you warning
reader beware

this writer
will
not
close
her book
again.

Was It Always Like This?

Was it always like this?
or did I have some days
even one day
free of you
wretched pain?

funny

I can't remember
any days of luxury
free
of you
wretched pain.

What was it like?
How did it feel
before I was
forced
into this circle
onto this wheel
of you

Have I always mapped
my future
including you

never knowing
if you
were coming
on vacation, too

Have I always lived
making plans
for a day
never knowing
when
I'd have
to put them away

Was it always like this?
how can I know?
my memories hold nothing
not full
of you

wretched pain.

August 11, 1985

Dear Mary,

I'm so happy finally to be writing my book. I've been very depressed these last few days, unable to listen to my favorite tapes or enjoy eating (you know I'm a mess when I can't eat happily), or do anything with joy. I've been reading a lot, as usual, even though this was the only thing I really wanted to do. Finally I even threw the books down.

It hit me that my depression was a way to hide my rage at not finding any way to write my story. You know, Mary, other people don't need to do this. They are happy to live their lives doing `normal' things, things I've never felt content doing. Now that I've started this, I feel peaceful. I'm even listening to Eric Clapton, something I haven't done for days. The tapes have been sitting on the floor next to my bed with this pad and pen. I finally picked them all up together.

I laugh because I know you're way out there in Arizona, not knowing the new life I've found in writing these pages to you. I guess you'll know soon enough. Will you be surprised?

I love you,
Linda

August 11, 1985

Dear Mary,

Did I ever take you to Roosevelt Island with me? Probably not, because that's the place I usually go to be alone. Anyway, the last time I was there, I was sitting on one of the benches near a fountain, reading. A lot of people ramble around there—families, bikers, runners—and the good thing about the place is that no one bothers me. It's a place to go when you want to be with people but you don't want any verbal contact.

The island has a ghastly statue of Teddy Roosevelt, with some of his famous sayings carved on huge slabs of concrete. Really, the place looks more like a cemetery; but sitting there makes me feel very much alive.

As I was sitting and reading, I heard a child coming along with his mom. He sounded very normal—laughing, chattering to her. Then I looked at him. He walked slowly, almost haltingly, avoiding stairs and inclines in his travels. As he came closer, I saw his little hands and I cringed. He had rheumatoid arthritis!

His mom kept urging him on. He would stare up at her as if to say, "You crazy or what?" He was only about two years old. How could this little guy explain his pain, when he didn't even know the words for it. He doesn't know other people feel different. He doesn't even understand what she is asking him to do—to "be normal."

My mind moved into his life. I named him Stevie—I always wanted to know someone with that name. I can see with wrenching clarity what's ahead for him. I see the day Stevie realizes he is different. I see him in first grade, at the playground, watching because he can't play. I see him watching while other kids try out for soccer and football. Maybe he can be team manager? Not likely. Why be reminded every day that you can't play?

I see him deciding—consciously or unconsciously—whether to function in society any way he can, or to be a depressed, wasted individual, rotting away in anger. I cry when I think of the choices his family will have to make because they have a "different" child, and how much they will influence the kind of person he will be. I know that if their influence is bad it could take Stevie's whole life and all his strength to break away from what they teach him.

Oh, Mary, as I watched him I grew so tired I could hardly hold my book. I laid it down and put my sunglasses on, hoping no one had seen my tears.

I love you,

Linda

Heavy Baggage

Sitting in the park
I see a boy
His walking is slow
and pained
I look at his face
and he's smiling.

He creeps
falteringly
closer
holding out hands
with crumpled joints
reaching for things
with a strange contorted grip.

All at once
lightning hits

his little hands
looks like mine.

"He's so tiny"
I cry to myself
barely holding on
to the bench.
A sick familiar
swell
sweeps into my stomach

the pounding in my chest
is so loud
I'm deafened.

Curiosity
turns to pain
knowing tears pour down my cheeks
legs so weak
I couldn't walk
if I tried

I know the life waiting
for this boy
so small

He carries baggage
that gets
heavier, harder to move
with each passing moment

And I can't help him
carry it.

August 11, 1985

Dear Mary,

Did I ever tell you how much I hate surgery? Four times in not even three years; I wonder how I've done it and come out emotionally alive. I want the cycle to stop. I want to be able to say, "STOP! I can't stand any more," and then all this madness would cease.

Such a nice fantasy. I would honestly rather have fantasies about something other than stopping the arthritis in my body, but it's my only priority.

Tell me, what do "normal" people fantasize about? Love? A new house? Life after death? I fantasize about life after surgery. I dream about how long my left hand can last before it goes under the knife again.

This brings up another point. I'm sick of hearing people tell me how well I'm doing. "Such strength," they sigh. I want to put a sign under my shirt,"BUZZ OFF," and when anyone says that to me I'll just blast them with the sign.

I would rather write "FUCK OFF" on the sign, but people would be so busy responding to the profanity, they'd miss the real point. Sometimes one has to compromise in life.

I do have a way of saying buzz off, though. I tune out. I smile a little sick smile and go off into me. I'm tired of doing that, too. Can I handle all these changes in me?

Mary, I don't like to be redundant, but I HATE SURGERY. I hate it so much I have to look it up in the dictionary every time I write it.

I love you,
Linda

Surgery Is Perjury

Surgery is
perjury
of the skin

Knives
take
a slice
of my life.

Needles
wheedle
out my blood.

Tourniquets
make me
want to call it
quits.

Saws
got me trembling
at the jaw

Blood vessels
turn
stomach
churns

In he goes
again
I lose
my second wind

Drugs
make me dry
but thank God
at least
I'm high

After two years
and four cuts
this gets to be
a rut.

Wrinkled and Worn

Wrinkled and worn
struggling inside
ripped
torn

feeling like
my life's
been shorn
with
Disease.

Tired of seeing it
feeling it

Looking good outside
till you find
the bumps

covered by clothes
seeming smooth
Strangers go by
knowing
they approve

does nothing
to give
me
a lift

Wrinkled and worn
weary
waiting
for the day life's cheery
at least
part of the time

People
seeing perfection
and other lies
of self-deception

People crave perfect
adore
beauty they can see

I resent my body's betrayal
of me.

July 1, 1985

August 11, 1985

Dear Mary,

Do you notice I start most of my letters with questions? I know now why I do that. I'm afraid to tell anyone anything unless I know people will be responsive. So I ask questions first, and if they respond, I go on. If they don't, I stop.

Is this my reaction to growing up in a family that can't interact? Am I not letting myself trust anyone because one unit of six people can't respond to each other in honesty?

This lack of trust is something I want to change. I want to sit down with our family and say, "let's chat," and have an honest, six-way conversation. I know I can't have that with anyone but you. So I've decided to find joy in what I do have. At least I have you. I know you respond, and others do, too. And when I get hurt by trusting and not getting a response, I have to learn to shrug and move on. There are lots of honest people in the world. I have to learn that it's okay to take a few lumps along the way. But most of all I have to learn to cherish what I have.

From now on, I'm going to try to start my letters with declarative statements, respecting the fact that you will respond to me, and you will do so honestly.

I love you,
Linda

August 11, 1985

Dear Mary,

There was an article in the paper this morning about handwriting analysis. For $12.00 I can copy a paragraph, sign it, and send it off to some guy (who is giving me a big break; it usually costs $100.00) and he will tell me all about my strengths and weaknesses.

Immediately I wanted to do it. I love it when other people tell me about myself. Oh, tell me, tell me, then I won't have to figure out me myself.

When I look in the mirror, I don't see what I see, I see what I think the world sees. I never judge me for myself. When an outsider says, "That looks good," then I like it, too. Or "Do something with your hair," makes me want to change it, right away.

My mirror isn't made of glass, it's made of the world's eyes.

Sadness is creeping up my legs.

I love you,
Linda

One Step Forward

I've got to
stop
trying to sing
in your key

stop my dreams
of living
through you
and live
through me

I'm on my way
forward,
but every now and then
I take a step
back
still
trying
to pack me into
you

It's a struggle
it's a climb
but this time I'm not
leaving
me
behind

When I'm standing
on my own,
living
in this mind
and this body

when I've finally
made my way
I'll be singing
in my key

But I'll never forget
the things
you gave
to me.

As Good As You

Can I sing?

Is it true
that I might really be as good
as you?

You see
I just never thought
I just never
knew that I

could
do anything
as well
as you.

You are the world
all others but
me

You have the
faith and the courage to be
who
and what you are

a singer

a writer

a dancer

a star

Can I sing?

It is really true

can I sing, too
as beautifully

as freely

as you?

August 11, 1985

Dear Mary,

I'm scared to write any more today.

This book is too honest.

I love you,

Linda

Where Is It?

Dishonesty

Please.
I want to call you my past.
I want you
                    at last
behind me.

Now I find myself
keeping in
          anger
          hurt
again.

Sheer dishonesty
why do you keep finding me?
Where can I hide from you
why do I hear your call?

What point do I prove
through you?

It's time...
How do I find it?
I want to lose
myself

in honesty.

August 7, 1985

August 11, 1985

Dear Mary,

As you can see, it's still August 11th. I can't stop writing. I'm like a tormented soul tied to this pen. But each time I put another word on this page, I'm less a maniac and I feel less pain.

I'm having a hard time with something and maybe you can help me figure it out. Why can't I be like other people? Why aren't I satisfied with the regular things in life? Why can't I accept what happens to me without questioning why, like others I've met with rheumatoid arthritis?

How often I've heard someone say, "I really don't know when this happened; I guess I just have to make the best of it." I'm talking about that kind of attitude not only toward illness, but in everything. My need for a different life is so deep and pervasive, I feel unable to contain myself and my illness.

Most of the time I accept this about myself, but sometimes, on days like today and moments like this second, I want to scream at myself, "Linda, just be regular!"

But I know I'm not. And those moments pass.

So do you have any ideas on why I can't be a typical Susie-kind-of-girl?

I love you,
Linda

A-Go-Go

My life
    for a word
that's never
been said

something space-age
untried
not soft and rumpled
like a worn-out bed.

I'm sick to death
of renovations
please god send me
a revelation.

My soul
for an upstart of verbiage
an unbeaten noun

all these words
they've been around
and around

Yes I plead for
an a-go-go thought
never wrought
with tears

what's this madness that's taken hold of me?

Now I see
I'm ushering in
my neoteric
sound
to be.

August 9, 1985

August 11, 1985

Dear Mary,

And another thing. I know I'm not dying with this disease. At least not physically. The slow kill, that's what I'm fighting. Building walls, brick by brick, air tight.

Because I don't want to think about it.

But I have to think about it because it makes me sicker not to think. I used to be able to kid myself about things like hang-gliding, skateboards, running, playing softball. I used to be able to say, "I don't care, I don't want to do that anyway. DAMN! How in hell do I know? I've had to say that to myself for so long I don't remember if my life was ever different.

Could I ever have done those things?

There's a big difference, Mary, between not doing something because you don't want to do it and not doing it because you can't. Where's the concept of "options," or "choices" for my life?

At times like these I feel very confused, as I did last July, on the night before my last surgery. I know there are others around me, in much worse shape than I am—dying, totally crippled.

I may have only partial choices, limited options, but some people have none at all. I'm one of the lucky ones. When I compare myself with all of humanity I feel better. Not happy that someone else is more racked up than I am, but happy that I can see some light in my own life.

I see my life and some of its tragedy, but I can also see its promise. It's like being asleep and awake at the same time; like a double vision that is so clear it obscures nothing. Because I see both up and down, bad and good. I see all points of view. Really, it makes me feel crazy sometimes.

I wonder briefly if you'll still love me after reading all this madness. The reply comes quickly—of course you will. That's why I'm writing to you.

I love you,

Linda

Pleasure and Pain

Hands
to grab with
to demand with
to pamper with gloves and rings,
and other silly things.

Hands
to give pain
to buckle in the rain
to teach me I'm human
every hour of the day.

Hands
to sew with
to sign `no' with
to write words with
to give me bliss

Hands
for using
confusing.

Hands using me
their pain
all can see.

Scars that heal
to be opened again
to hurt so much
but to be my friends

The deepest pain
the highest pleasure
how many, countless,
treasures
I have made
with these

Hands

All I ask
stop hurting now
please.

Insane

Writing words
anger escapes
no happy lines
no happy pieces
tonight.

Looking ahead
to weeks of pain
my body
convulses with
disdain.

Months again of people's stares
at the way I'm forced to bare
my life.

Words taste
bitter
Anger swells
No ringing
of life's bells
tonight.

Still I love this life of mine
on nights like this
sanity
is
dismissed.

Words of passion
thoughts of pain
this past year has been
running
constant
rain

And yet I'm willing
continuing
to live with life
On nights like this
I feel
insane.

August 11, 1985

Dear Mary,

I've been thinking a lot about "the one that won't go away." The arthritis attack, that is.

As soon as I put that sentence on paper my mind blanked.

God it hurts to see it in writing. Yes, there is a possibility it could happen. Again. Of course, I could also walk out of my house tomorrow and get hit in the head with a flying brick. But my chances for an RA attack are much higher.

Anyway, it terrifies me, because I think I'd probably kill myself or something stupid like that. Why do I worry about something that hasn't happened? Because it almost did. Last October I started an arthritis attack that lasted from Halloween till March. It's the first one I've had that went on so long; it's the first one that lasted more than three days. All I could think about was making it through the day, so I could go home and sleep.

People I met at that time believed I was a late sleeper, not very interested in life. One man I dated briefly told me he thought I was lazy. (You can see why I dated him briefly!) What do people who hurt like that all the time go through? Lazy? Uninterested? Uninteresting? Antisocial? How about sick, tired, and in excruciating pain for starters, then we can move on to fed up, isolated, angry, hopeless. For the first time in my life, I asked to die.

This is too hard. I'm going to take a shower. Maybe I can finish this later.

I love you,
Linda

The One That Doesn't Leave

Nightmares
circle me

teasing

of the life
that may
some day
            own me
            be mine.

to lie down
and not
            be able
to rise again.

I keep searching for the sin I've committed
to earn
such torturous
dreams.

Will I be able
to go on
            only
in my mind?

or will this be
a state
I'm not inclined

to survive?

I won't know,
            will I,
until it hits.

August 11, 1985

Dear Mary,

Hi. It's me again. The shower helped hide the sounds of my tears from the others at home. It felt good to let them fall.

Yes, Mary, I asked to die. More than once. That's what severe continuous pain does to me. Now I know. To take a whole Percodan (before the attack I had only taken a quarter at a time) and feel my pain only narrowly chipped. I don't know how I came out of those months clean of drugs.

What was it that made me go on?

To compound the situation, I had my third surgery during that time. To get my left hand strong enough so I could have more surgery on my right hand. Dressing myself with one hand in all that PAIN!

Why did I go on?

When the pain began to ease, I tortured myself with the thought that it would be back, any minute. It really was no way to live! Even when I knew the pain was physically subsiding, it was still with me mentally. But something inside me said, "Time—time will help erase it."

And it has somewhat. But still, every time I don't feel well, I say, "This is it. It's here again and it's here to stay."

I'm working on this because if I continue this train of thought each time I feel funky, I'm nuts for sure. It's the hardest work I've ever done.

I love you,

Linda

When Thursday Comes Again

My feet

on Thursday
to move
took
all my might.

On Saturday
my feet
took flight.

On Monday

they

walked two miles
with me in tow.

But how can I know

when Thursday
will come
again?

August 11, 1985

Dear Mary,

I've been reading a book called, *In the Belly of the Beast*, by Jack Abbott. He's a man who spent most of his life in jail. I'd love to write to him or someone like him and discuss what it's like to be in that kind of prison,— one not imposed on you by your own body, but by other men. The things he has gone through—put himself through—made me cry, shuddering at the ways of man.

Somehow, I've made comparisons between his life and the lives of people with diseases they can't escape. It's very different, yet somehow the same.

When a prisoner is released from incarceration, he's confused, really not knowing how to act in society. He's been away for so long; maybe he never learned how to behave like everybody else in the first place. If my disease left me, it would take years for me to adjust to health. Oh, to be able to spend my money on health and not on fighting disease! To spend my time on health instead of trying to reach it! To be accepted in the world for my health instead of having to prove myself in spite of it!

I feel guilty making these comparisons. Anyone reading this in prison would probably laugh at the thought of me comparing my life to theirs.

Well, I've done it. I've come right out and compared chronic illness to a prison. Maybe by finally doing that, I've begun to set myself free.

I love you,
Linda

Deceived

I was born
like any other

had two legs
arms
and all the body parts
any child needs
to make her start
in life.

Slowly it began
to dawn on me
the body
I had
wasn't meant
for regularity.

I had been
lied to
deceived.

Anger raged through me
pouring out
at its whim
yes

I was deceived
by life
who'd have believed
this fate
would
happen
to me?

August 11, 1985

Dear Mary,

I've just reread what I wrote to you today. I cried again with each letter. Half with pain and anger, half with joy that I have someone I can write to. I guess I should have realized there was someone to write to all along. That's nice to know after 30 years. The pain and anger come from knowing how well qualified I am to write this book. I wish I weren't the right person for this job.

See you tomorrow.

I love you,
Linda

August 12, 1985

Dear Mary,

It's been a rough day. Last Saturday afternoon I slid down a few stairs. Happening to anyone else it would have been nothing, but for my body it was a major calamity. All day long I visualized someone grabbing me by the hair and slamming me against a concrete wall. I kept asking myself what I possibly could have done during any of my lifetimes to deserve such pain.

I guess I have to remind myself that this is the only life I know and it isn't—hasn't been—fair. When I look at life that way I stop searching for someone to blame it on. And I don't feel as anxious.

Having plans and then cancelling them has become an accepted part of my life. I used to hate it, and I did whatever I wanted in spite of the pain, making myself sicker. Now I stop cold and cool out. This whole week has been cancelled, knocked off the calendar.

But losing this one will make next week so much sweeter.

I love you,
Linda

I Like It When It Works

Body like mine
with so may quirks
I like this body
but only when it works.

Grumbles and cracks
from feet all up my back
but when it's time
to dance
body kicks back
to let me prance.

Mind starting off
slowly each day
giving me fire
to speed
farther
and farther away
from the life
my body tries
to bind me to.

I'll be back for you,
body
on the days you want
to move

check you out...
But carry no doubt
this mind's
not waiting around for you.

A body's fine
swimming in time
climbing a little here
and there..
Yes, most of the time
doing its share
But I've come to care
only
when it works.

But work or not
after giving you all this thought
moving on
because my world
is won
with or without
you.

Making my choice
and

liking it when
it works.

No more tailoring
life
to
its
quirks.

August 13, 1985

Dear Mary,

We have two parents who love us very much. They just don't say it in the "regular" way.

I've never heard either of them say the words, "I love you," to anyone, have you? They say it through the act of providing. All this has made me angry for a long time—all my life. I would have died to hear either of them say those three words. Is it the passage of time or the futility of waiting that lets me put that fantasy to rest?

I've given up ever trying to live in their house. It's never felt right to me, living there. I'm not sure it even feels right for them.

For whatever reason, they are still not ready to speak. Feelings are so terrifying they don't even attempt to talk about them. Who am I to change them? I'm only accountable for me, and I better get moving. I can only take along those who are willing to get in the car and ride.

Life with our parents always left me gasping for more air. I'm still not getting any air from them, but now there are others to open those windows. I'll turn to them now and love them for who they are and what they give me.

It has helped me enormously to write my feelings about my life with our parents. My poems are sad. Angry. But they stand as written, because they're my feelings. I'm not just going to allow myself to have those feelings, but to express them.

I love you,
Linda

We Still Have a Chance

We had
all
the right
people.

Owned all
the right things.

But most of all
love
was there
is here.

Can we learn
to let
our love meet,

not pass,
strangers walking
on opposite sides
of the street?

Yes, we love each other.
How much longer
will it take
for us
to discover
the way
to let it
be known.

For I'm not blaming you,
I hold the guilty heart
as heavy
as it is true.

Finding a way
grabbing any chance
to be
at peace
with you.

An Open Letter to You

To Julie

I would hold you in a minute

go to the edge and beyond
but our bond
was silence

I can hold it
no longer.

To call
is to hear
lots of ummms and ohhhs
what
really happens
seems not for me
to know.

Even the letters
you said would come
one
full of pain
was yours to me
was mine to you

one moment
one fleeting moment
it seemed we had
a connection

other than
our face.

How can
I tell you
How can
I let you know

It's time
for us
to open
the years—the door
that shut
between us.

How can I
tell you
that door has a key
How can I tell you
It's time
for you and me
to grow.

I Needed You to Water Me

My father
waters plants
instead
of me

He turns the soil
instead
of turning me.

All the seasons
he never saw
heard
felt
my need.

Why does it feel
so new
that now
whatever my father may say
or do

I don't care.

My father...
His daughter has
a story
he'll never read.

My father
thought
his duty
was only
to plant
the seed.

The Audition

How was
the audition?

She didn't listen—I'm not
an actress;
I never tried out
I never said anything
about
an audition.

Did you perform
well?

She's got the wrong daughter.
It wasn't me
Can't she tell
which one I am?

Did you memorize
your lines?

She's not even looking
I'm losing my footing

I look at her
and think about
the part I didn't get

The audition that failed
was mine, for her

I cringe
and things begin to blur
the throb increases

And I understand about the big one—
the audition
that never ceases.

7-27-85

August 13, 1985

Dear Mary,

My body and I feel better today, but we're still scared of tomorrow. The fear is different now. It doesn't stop me from living, from starting new things because I'm not sure I'll be able to finish. Even on days I feel the worst, I move around mentally, spiritually. That's what has given me freedom

Oh, I can breathe deeply when I read that sentence.

Assimilating the concept of cycles into my existence has also encouraged my vision. Although I'm afraid of tomorrow, I'm ready for it, because I know there's also a day after tomorrow. And that day may be sweet!

Do you have thoughts like this? What are your fears? How do you work through them?

I love you,
Linda

August 13, 1985

Dear Mary,

It's time for me to be doing something I love, something that makes me feel like singing each morning as I prepare myself for the day ahead. Time for me to sit down and write some more.

I'm not sure why this is such a change in my life. All work is expression. I'd love to have expression without responsibility, but I know that's out. I'm too guilty. Taking care of other people, as in teaching—I can't do that any more.

Writing is great fun, but who gets paid for writing whatever they want? Very few people. Right now that's my goal—to get paid for writing—and I'm working toward it. Maybe by age 60 I'll sell something. I know one thing; now that I've started expressing myself through writing, I won't stop. It used to make me sick, trying to express myself. Now I get sick if I don't.

Some kind of fear made me stop before. Would I get a good evaluation or be judged a lousy writer? People are able to squelch each other through that kind of intimidation.

You know better than anyone else how much I always wanted to please. Any time I expressed myself honestly, someone got mad.

Did I think they would kill me? Maim me for life? Possible but not probable. It's hard for me to face the fact that I've been such a chicken! But I have. And now that I've faced it, it's even harder to admit it. But I'm doing that, too.

Honest expression. Doing what I love. I'm excited.

I love you,
Linda

August 13

Dear Mary,

I've been asked more than a few times how I feel about missing parts of myself, having scars. Do I feel like a woman who is missing a breast, a man who loses a limb? I'm always surprised to be hit with this one.

Because I happen to have scars on very visible parts of my body I am forced to deal with anyone who sees them and wants to comment, or to share a weird view of life. I've even been asked, in the middle of Bloomingdale's, if I had tried to commit sucide! (That person was really out of it; the scars are on the wrong side of my wrists.) Whatever other people's fantasies, I have to live through their comments.

The first thought I have on this is: what gives anyone the right to comment on my life, my body, without my invitation to do so? Because I have a disease that makes me different, I'm a dumping ground for other people's fears in life—that they'll get a disease that won't go away. I have to hear about poor Aunt Betty, Stella down the street, and on and on.

I'm not talking about friends. I'm talking about acquaintances and total strangers.

Getting to the next point: how do I feel about missing parts of myself—the four joints in my right hand, for instance. This gets very complicated. I flash back to the reasons why I had the surgery in the first place. Did all this agony serve the purpose I wanted it to? But that's another question entirely. So back to the one I don't want to answer. See, I even try to bluff myself in writing!

My original parts hurt. A lot. They were swollen, red, achy. I'm glad they're gone. But I wish the new parts worked better.

I've always loved new things, because they work better than the old stuff. That's not necessarily so with joints. But they don't hurt. That's the key. I still feel attractive. The skin is soft.

I feel whole.

Now to the third question: how do I feel about scars? Four scars, to be exact. People are funny about scars. Some people see mine and come running up to show me theirs. Camaraderie, I guess. Sometimes they want to one-up me "You think yours are bad—take a look at mine," spoken in a booming voice.

Scars leave me wide open. Hands are such an elementary part of life—people use them all the time, right out in the open. I would have preferred the scars under my bikini line; but hey, there's no arthritis there. I don't like "people" knowing that I've been "through something." They tend to get curious about what it was I "went through." Frankly, it's a pain in the ass.

I have a few standard answers to the question, "What happened to your hand?" depending on how it's asked. Some of my favorites are:

What happened to your face?

It's an old war wound.

My sister cut me with a knife. (Sorry, Mary.)

I have rheumatoid arthritis and plastic joints. Don't feel sorry for me or I'll slap you.

Get the gist? Hostile, right? I'm just so tired of it.

More on this later.

I love you,
Linda

August 14, 1985

Dear Mary,

I had some extremely interesting conversations at NIH today. One was with a crazy man who wore pot holders for earrings, hooked onto his ears with rubber bands. (They didn't even match his dress.) The other was with a 78-year-old woman who had the most deformed hands I'd ever seen. None of her fingers moved in the same direction. There was no support from one joint, one tendon to the next. Each moved independently, leaving this woman in total frustration.

As we sat and chatted, we began a debate on whether other people can possibly be aware of what we go through—everything from the fear of losing movement and life as we know it, to the pain of every moment. At first I agreed with her. No, there's no way anyone could possibly be aware of this pain without living through it.

Then I began to think—what about the person prone to headaches? Sore throats? bladder infections? anything? Most people know about temporary pain. Suppose I asked someone to visualize her occasional, interfering malady as a constant in her life.

I think an understanding of the insidious nature of chronic problems is available to just about anyone who is human. However, I do think it requires a lot of visualization. And a lot of reminding.

I love you,
Linda

August 14, 1985

Dear Mary,

There are many kinds of pity. Some are sympathetic, while other kinds are patronizing. Sometimes I listen to how I feel when someone is speaking—does his voice make me want to cringe or does it bring tears to my eyes and make me want to give him a hug?

Some people look at me and speak to me as if they are fearful of catching "it." I don't think they are even sure what "it" is. A lot of people eliminate the need for understanding by saying, "Oh, you do so well." And then there are the few who know just how to handle "it" and me.

There is something I want from people. And that is the understanding that I can do a job, run a home, socialize as well as anyone else. Except sometimes. Sometimes I can't. And that's ok. Just like any other human being who, from time to time, has troubles of any sort.

Some day I may have to alter that "sometimes" to "often." But I've decided not to worry about that. It wears me out to be so concerned for my future. What I really want is to get through the next 24 hours without any patronizing leers. Just a little understanding of two important words: "human" and "different."

I love you,
Linda

Courageous, They Say

(Read with a nagging voice)

You take it SO well
You're SO
Courageous

How do you DO it?

What light do you see?

I could NEVER do it—
thank God
I'M only stuck with me.

My life is SO different
Things are TRULY swell
I'm EVER so happy
Really.
Can't you tell?

To DRAW such a card
Your life seems SO
hard
Well, at least mine's not bad
I hardly EVER feel sad
Like you.

But dear, you're SO
Courageous
Too bad
you're always
going through those stages.

Hey, I can put up with it.
I'll shuffle through
those pages
of life
with you

But ME
thank God
I only get the flu.

August 16, 1985

Dear Mary,

Perfect. Obsessed with being, looking, feeling perfect—or as close as possible. It's a trap! "Normal" people have a hard enough time living up to the ideal, let alone the ones playing without a full deck.

It's always amazed me, this battle for perfection; and how many times have I found myself caught up in it? Often. We all know life is anything but perfect—we are anything but perfect.

I've never minded that people try to look, feel as good as possible. It's part of our responsibility to ourselves. But there's so little space for people who are different—and that small space is very crowded.

I hear on the news that children with cancer, some without limbs or hair, can go to camps where they'll feel "normal"—where they can take off their wigs and their artificial limbs and feel better about themselves. Would this be necessary if the rest of the world held a little space open for them? If we would let them be different, right where they are, who-ever they're with? Maybe. I'm not sure.

PEOPLE ARE ALL THE SAME.

We all breathe, sweat, urinate, live, die. I wish we'd give up this sham of holding irregularities away from us, as far as possible, as if physical and mental differences smelled funny. As though, if you got close enough, you'd catch them.

If there were a place where we, I, all of us could just be as good as we are, life would be cake. And all our differences could be the frosting.

I love you,

Linda

No Typos Please

Letter perfect
No typos
Please
Check it once
then
Check it again
Go over life
With a fine-tipped
pen.

Get the White-Out
the correction tape
It's got
to be
Perfect
for Pride's
Precious
Sake.

Erase the smudges
Center the title
Margins
in sync
It must read
smoothly
not to cause
a blink.

Errors
maybe
in the center
But not
on the surface.

We know
what's
inside,
but never
never
admit

Imperfect.

August 17, 1985

Dear Mary,

I've been writing for ten years—short stories, poems, songs, letters to you. Not steadily though, only when I had an arthritis attack. There are moments, hours during an attack when the pain is so bad. Pain killers only slightly numb the contortions jolting my body. In that half-awake state, I find myself composing.

For hours I lie there in the dark and make rhymes that twist and turn. I memorize each one before moving on to the next. The next morning, or a few days later, I write down everything I created during the attack. Then I take it to a wastebasket and dump it in.

I used to feel like a bulemic, letting myself be consumed by words, then relentlessly throwing them out. I hid my writing from everyone, including myself. I couldn't tolerate my own expression. When I think of the reams of paper with my words that I have trashed, sadness sweeps through me; sorrow so strong my guts throb.

Then on May 30 of this year, something slapped hope into me. Two days before, a major attack had knocked me out. The usual scenario occurred, even the rain tapping on my window as I composed my poems. I got up on the 30th and typed it all down. Then I went to the wastebasket—and I just couldn't, couldn't throw it out!

And then the real miracle happened. I reread the ten or twelve poems and the children's book I had written, and I must have cried enough for a million years. I cried for all the books, poems, stories, letters, pieces of myself I threw away.

I cried for everything I've been through and everything I've put myself through. But most of all I cried because I had finally allowed my own eyes to read the expressions created by the brain behind them. I've always wanted my eyes to hide the brain they window, never wanted them to meet. Never let the world see them working together. I was sure that my thoughts weren't worthy of paper, but I could never stop them. Even though I threw them away, the next time around, the words crowded out again, and again.

Now I can't stop writing. Sometimes I feel ill and want to scream "enough!" But the words don't stop. Sometimes I want to feel blank again, because I'm so overwhelmed with all those words and my need to get them out. I guess that's what happens when you try to erase ten years. The piles of paper just get higher. I roll over in bed and land on a pen, a piece of crumpled paper.

I know I'm still censoring myself, because I'm scared of what hasn't been said.

I love you,
Linda

Rain

Rain
Is so right tonight

As I put out my light

With part of a pill.

Rain
that makes me feel
At peace
Is with me
at least
Until dawn

Hitting the window
the watery sound
Allows me the freedom
to lie around

Rain
while I'm healing

Ease
is what I'm feeling
No need to please

Rain
As I'm healing.

That Blanked-Out Feeling
or
Hiding the Monster From Me

I feel trite

Words seem banal
tonight

Writing fluffs of nothing
There's ink on this paper
but it's the
disappearing kind.

It seems I get
like this
When the world isn't
with me.
I can't sit
peer at it
here
In the palm of my hand

All I see is blank
running to the dock
sure my ship just
sank.

Nothing seems worth it
I feel less than alive
unimportant
in a world that's bare

This blankness used to get me
off the hook.
Looking at
nothingness
I didn't have to share
my feelings
with me.

Then maybe the hurt
Would go away
Damn!
why doesn't emptiness
Pay
for me
any more?

Not Tonight—I Have a Headache

No more
I'm not writing
any more words
tonight

My brain
is beat
Inside
and
Out

From grabbing you
pen
Reaching for you
paper

Exhausted
I plead
No more!
Not tonight!
I have a headache
and
no end's
in sight

to this constant
barrage of titles
and rhymes

words
flow fast
and easy
but tonight
I'd rather
Leave them
behind

Eyelids
drooping
Lower lip
in a pout

oh God
Not one more line tonight!
let me put
out
this light.

Fast-Moving Potion

It's not life's
looks
but its speed
that's laughing hard
haunting me

It's not the shape
it's the motion
My days have taken
a fast-moving potion

Time is like a bullet
blowing in and out
my gut

Time I've wasted
slaps my moving sides
I'm unable to ignore
time
I've let erode
before

It's not the sun
it's the moon
that has me gaping
          open
          wounded.

Today
    tomorrow
are my sun
but yesterday's
waste
has me
under the gun.

August 17, 1985

Dear Mary,

Now that I've let my past catch up with me it seems that time is mocking me, moving with lightning speed. Time is saying to me "You better get it all down! What a waste of time you've been." I'm running, leaping, passing myself at every bend but time keeps pounding me with its urgency.

I was never aware of it before I started writing, started expressing, started actually keeping my work. Now I feel minutes chasing me and I better move my ass.

I see myself open from head to toe. It's as if someone took a razor-sharp knife, started at my forehead and just slit me right down the middle. Oozing all over every step I take. Oozing with words.

But no matter how time wants to taunt me, I'm not closing up again. Staying open is the only way to save this body.

I love you,
Linda

Boxed Sides Now Open

Boxed sides

Glued in

Learned how
to slit me open
with a pen

Lid shut

Slammed down

No one around
no help to be found
only within

Boxed sides
punching out
instead of
scrunching in

Pushing out
the sides
instead of
pushing
further
   in

Steps to climb
stumbling around
on paper
with a pen.

Never again

boxed in.

August 17, 1985

Dear Mary,

But all this is driving me crazy. Driving down the street, pulling over to find a pen before I scream. Staying home instead of playing because I want to write. When will the pile be high enough?

Friends are rolling their eyes, "putting up" with me, I think with just a little jealousy. My body is cooperating, moving along with my brain. Even if it doesn't, I know I won't throw out my pages again.

As people speak to me, their eyes, the way their noses move give me ideas. I feel like an idiot saying, "Will you move exactly that way again; you just gave me an idea for a poem." But I do it. And they know I'm nuts. A maniac in three months! A monster on the loose.

But how does the word HAPPY hit you? Hee Hee.

I love you,
Linda

Hold On

Hold on!
I've got to
write you down

Stop everything!
don't mind me
I'm only looking
for a pencil
some paper
I have to
write down
one more
link
to me.

Pull over to that drugstore
I just ran
out of ink.

Don't worry
We won't be too late
but
If I can't write this down
I won't be able
to think.

What did you say?
I was lost
in a thought
that needed
to be put down on paper.

No, I'm not ignoring you.
Yes, I'll get over this craziness
soon
(Maybe ten years or so).
until then...

Hold on...Stop the show..
I've only got a few
words to go

I don't mean to drive you nuts
But

hand me that paper
It's time to
strut
my words.

August 19, 1985

Dear Mary,

Let me tell you about my day. First I went to acupuncture and spent $40.

Then I drove to the nutritionist to find out what vitamins and minerals I need and what foods I'm allergic to, and to learn that I have "stomach dumping syndrome." Altogether, I dropped $240.00 there.

Then I headed to NIH to be heated up and twisted around for about an hour and a half.

Now, doesn't all that sound like fun? You're lucky you're not around. I'm in a bad mood, broke, and have a headache from taking ten vitamins at dinner. Other than that, things are great.

Oh, and by the way, I start work tomorrow.

I love you,
Linda

August 20, 1985

Dear Mary,

I never understood why people drank, got high, whatever. But the thought of crawling off somewhere, depressed and hooked on drugs, is beginning to have some appeal. Things are always so clear to me—pain—people in pain. It's beginning to tear at me.

At NIH today, some other patients and I were joking about the things we go through: the craziness we put up with from other people, and how hard we are on ourselves. We were laughing as we shared our tales of horror. How did we learn to laugh at such things in life—especially the things that happen to us? I think it's a Joni Mitchell song that says, "Laughing and crying—it's the same release." I think she's right.

Today, at this moment, I'm sick of knowing how crystal clear life is—the good and the bad. I'd like a little shelter from reality, some long-term fantasy to call my own.

I love you,
Linda

Hand Me Some Haze

I don't want
to see it clearly
`cause then it doesn't
bother me.

Get me a little
   haze
Blow it around some
I can't take
this town
bright and clear.

How about a beer
Hand me a pill
It's the only way
to get
a thrill
living in this town.

It's hard as hell
   and
I'm down
but there's still
   a chance
If I can become
unclear.

Take me to a movie
a fantasy
Keep the lights down low
'cause I don't even want to
   know
if it's still daylight.

Leave me alone
unless
you can come up
with a way
to help me keep
   out
the sight of day

Keep it off
turn it low
   `cause I don't even want to know.

September 1, 1985

Dear Mary,

Another frequent inquiry I get is "How serious is it?"

Last weekend I went to a party. I was cutting myself a piece of cheese, when a woman sitting next to me asked the popular opening question: "What's wrong with your hand?" Six or seven other people sitting in the vicinity all stopped talking and looked. I almost said "I'm dying of a serious disease and you can catch it," but I tactfully moved to the second reply on my list: "I had surgery."

Hoping the conversation was over, I turned to talk to my friend, but the woman asked again. So I told her I had rheumatoid arthritis. Then came, "So, how serious is it?" I asked myself, "Does this woman really think I want to share this information with her? Is she always this rude?"

I peered inside myself and asked "How serious is it, Linda?" I played the conversation back and forth in my head, realizing what a packed question that was: serious according to whom? People who aren't walking? People who are more or less healthy? Doctors? Me?

Finally I came back to reality and saw her assessing the situation for herself. With a last look at me, she said, "Yes, it must be serious. And I thought I had problems." As she turned to walk away, I noticed she had no left arm.

I love you,

Linda

A Matter Of Degree

Is it serious?
It's a matter of degree.
Who's making the judgement,
You, or me?

Are we deciding
On a Wednesday?
or a Thursday?

Let's decide on
    Friday.
It's easier
for me to say.

    Or

Maybe we should
wait until spring.
My body feels better
when the birds
and the lovers
                sing.

How serious....
  a man dying of cancer?
  a baby born with no fingers?

How serious....
  a question that lingers
  long after it's asked

Who's to say?
Who's to know?

It's a concept
that comes and goes.

September 29, 1985

Dear Mary,

I haven't written for a month. Reading over this pile of stuff again, I know why I tried to ignore it. It makes me cry. The way I manage to hide my pain away amazes me. Could I live through it if I always allowed myself to be aware? No. I couldn't.

A person with an open sore on her face tries her best to heal it. How do I heal the open sores of my heart? Do I even have a heart? Sometimes I feel I've become so hard. Some days I look in the mirror and I'm shocked by the hardness in my eyes. "That can't be my face, my jaw set so tight." So you see, even when I think I've forgotten what has happened to me, just put it away, it shows.

Where's the hammer? Maybe I can pound the pain out of me.

I love you,
Linda

Where's the Middle?

I don't think of
what I've been through
the hours of pain
known to few.

I march, head high
eyes feeling scratchy
forbidden to cry.

A body
  a mind
held so rigid
  so tight
even hiding from myself
the years of my plight.

Meeting each day
acting in this play
that life is kind

When the truth
that's landed on me
is far from sweet.

Feeling confused.

Do I sit
        stew
            brood?
ignore
      evade
this life I'm walking through?

The answer lies somewhere
  between
    rage
  and blankness

The road reaching home feels
so thankless
two steps ahead
  teetering in the middle
two steps behind

praying for balance.

September 30, 1985

Dear Mary,

I'm walking the halls of NIH this morning feeling pretty spunky when all of a sudden Fred wheels by. We walk together, me on my own two feet, he on his own two wheels. Fred and I used to sit together in occupational therapy and compare progression, regression, moans, etc.

As we moved along, I realized that the kinds of things we chatted about were not your mundane everyday subjects, but there we were, carrying on as if the topic was what to have for lunch.

I'm noticing more and more how weird it is to treat being a patient at NIH , in- or out-, like brushing your teeth.

I'm still confused about where the center is. Damn, I thought I had that figured out yesterday.

I love you, I think,
Linda

October 2, 1985

Dear Mary,

At NIH today, I was pushing Fred to the elevator in his wheelchair. (What was I doing that for? I have no business doing that.) Anyway, Fred said to me, "You know, your hands really are noticeable, but only if you point them out." And I wondered out loud whether I actually go around pointing them out.

Do I?

I love you,
Linda

October 3, 1985

Dear Mary,

I had a dream last night. There I was standing in this huge basement. Directly ahead of me were a washer and dryer, and a load of dirty laundry.

So what did I do? I started the laundry. Just when I had that first pile under control, I turned and saw four more washers and dryers and four more piles of dirty clothes. A woman came down once in a while to check on how I was doing.

There I stood. Doing a mountain of everyone else's laundry. Not one damn piece of it was mine.

I love you,
Linda

October 7, 1985

Dear Mary,

The season is changing. We are again moving into October. At the end of this month last year, I was descending into my six-month depression. It was during that six months that I decided to live. Of course, I wasn't able to say the word depression. I stated it in physical terms: "My body is killing me." "I can't move." "My arthritis is the worst it's ever been."

When I'm depressed, I get sick. It's about time I found another way to deal with depression. I want to be able to say, "I'm depressed because...." Instead, I get an ulcer. I get rheumatoid arthritis. Why can't I learn other ways to scream for help? I'm trying. I'm learning.

I love you,
Linda

October 8, 1985

Dear Mary,

I can't help it, I keep writing about the same old topic: Every time I hurt anywhere, I'm sure this is it. What happened to me this time last year will happen again and I'll be in a wheelchair trying to get the strength to kill myself.

Then I go through a process of realization—talking to myself—remembering that I did get better. And the more I allow myself verbal expression, the better I feel. So I always come to the conclusion, "If I express myself as well as I can, take care of myself and love myself, that's all I can ask of me." And I'm trying so hard to do all of those things. My life is finally falling into place.

I pray for the day I don't waste one minute thinking of what could happen to me, and just live the day I have.

I love you,
Linda

Cycles

A mind
  of cycles

Questions
  answers
all the same
persuasion.

I know
the cycle will always
  be
    me.

But can I learn to make it
grow smaller
turn faster
in my mind

Then I won't
be plagued
by
  this
    waste of time

Time
that could be
productive
  and lively
  and free of the worry
  the torment
  the terror

of what my
      tomorrows might be.

October 9, 1985

Dear Mary,

One thing that helps me through the cycle I've been telling you about is the fact that I now know that there are people who are willing to help me, any way they can. I never believed this before. People were always there, but I never wanted to depend on them. I thought we would all fail. Nothing could be done. My situation was hopeless and all I could do was wait for whatever fate decided to hand me.

Yes, I went to the doctor, got my shots, did all the things a good patient should. One thing was missing—my participation in the way my life was going. If I did participate, it was negative. My health was "his problem." He was a disappointment, because he couldn't find a cure for me. The angrier I got, the less responsibility I felt for my own health. The result was a sick, angry Linda with nothing and no one to believe in.

And where was "God" in this mess? I cried "Not fair," which is true. I backed myself into a corner with a barbed-wire fence around my life. No one could get in and I couldn't get out.

I'm finally learning to trust people, letting them help me, but it's hard. Hard giving up all those feelings that helped keep me ill mentally as well as physically. Those feelings were what I knew, and somehow, I got something out of perpetuating them. It's hard to let go. Some of the people I fought with before stuck with me, and will continue to do so. It's up to me to see that and learn to believe in them.

I love you,
Linda

You Always Knew It
(To Dr. Brandt)

You told me
over
and
over again

"You're special"

I never felt it
never knew.
But I liked
the way
I saw myself
through you.

Now I sense it!
Special's
coming
around

It's sprinkled
about my hair,
reflecting
in my eyes

The feeling's coming
from within
and I'm trying it on
for size.

Finally

I agree.
It's true!
How did you know?

You knew
before I could ever
see.

Now I dance
I bask
in this bright
shining light
that is me.

To D.L.

(To Dr. Goldstein)

On
Off
More
Less
Sleepy
Uneasy
Hooked
Clean
Someone helping in between
pills.

Bonnie Thornton Says.....

Up!
Out!
Make a fist!
I'll give you a list
of what
to do.

You can lift
two ounces
of anything
and all the air
you like

but don't you dare
do more than that.

Push!   Harder!
Give me more!
Those climbing percentages
are what I adore.

Whatever you do
don't
let it drift—

I'll show you
how
to lift
that pen
for life

Bonnie Thornton says

O.T.
It's the biggest trip
It's the only way
to get
a grip

Bonnie, by the look
of my hand
You don't have to say it
again.

I'll do whatever
Bonnie Thornton
says
I'll follow
Bonnie's rules

She's giving me
back
those precious tools

my hands.

Needles Galore

(To Bob Shapero)

Those needles
they send me
through
the floor.

It's needles
needles

needles
galore

In my toes
the middle of my chin
my hands
my wrists
where haven't they been?

The jolt
is electric
cosmic
and mean
Is it a wonder
Is it deranged
that often I dream

of needles
needles
needles galore.

Needles
needles
Give me some more

Of that strange
juice
that pumps through me
as you slide the needle
in
and turn it
like a key.

An Image of Mary

Mary
Some of the things
you've helped me get through

are they only in my mind
or are they true?

Truth or image
my vision of you
has given me space
to live anew.

With you
it's safe to cry
With you

it's hard to lie
about the things
that happen
to me.

I don't care
if you live
the way
you teach others to be.

I care only
selfishly
of the now
you seem to have given
me.

Mary
are you an image?
are you true?
The one thing I'm sure
of

is my love
for you

October 9, 1985

Dear Mary,

Another thing that has helped me is my refusal to put up with non-communication. It's amazing what I used to go through to have a "relationship." Anyone wants a relationship with me now, we both put out—whether it's family, friend, or lover. Or nothing!

This helps me feel clearer, more in control. It's as if I have a part, a little input into the world around me. If I have to lose friends, family, lovers, I will. I hope not, but I will risk it. The life I lived before was not working for me. It never did. I've been sick since I was seven years old.

Maybe it's time to change.

I love you,
Linda

I Hate Fiction

Predictions
acts of fiction.
I'm tired
of second guessing

your thoughts

your moves

I want fact
"like it is"
no maybes,
sort ofs,
we'll sees,

wanting to know
for sure
what's in it
for
me.

Hold on
hang on
just a little longer

feeling naked
open
on all sides

tired
of this merry-go-round.
I want off
this
ride

Tell me for sure
no changing
your mind
don't
give me that stuff
about being in a
bind.

You're putting me
off
with this game
of wait-and-see

I'm about to go off
and find
a stable
secure
non-fiction

life
for
me.

October 10, 1985

Dear Mary,

A strange thing is happening to me. I want a home, for the first time in my life. Before, the thought of having a home of my own made me gag. I lived in houses, in apartments. But they've never felt like part of me. I was just a wandering body, with a mind unattached.

Now I long for a place for me, a place that shows in the furnishings I choose, the flowers I arrange, the colors of who I am and what I want my life to say. I want to decide, yes, I like that color for my drapes. No, I don't want that on my walls.

And when it's all finished, I'll know the minute I walk inside that it's mine.

I love you,
Linda

I Want a Home

Home
Walls that I
own

Where are you?

Now that I
feel you in my insides
I want you
for my outsides,
too.

I don't want to get you
through a
man
or a parent's dollar

I want you
  through
    me

Through the sweet
        sweat
of my collar

Where are you
I want you
Now

I'll give up other
    things
    I want
for you
somehow

I want
a home
to clutter.

October 11, 1985

Dear Mary,

When is a book finished? When it's time to put it down and start another. My pain is lessening and going away.

Writing this has helped me through the hardest, but most satisfying part of my life.

This book is a tribute to my own feelings. It's certification that I have them, that they are real and no one can take them away, including myself, ever again.

I love you,
Linda

Subsiding Pain

The pages of books
I didn't remember
choosing to read

used to turn
almost
without me

in an unattached
uneventful way.

Then
in October
I started to be
involved
in the title
introduction
and body
of every book,

wanting
to start at the beginning
and read each word again.

Then I panicked
there were too many books
too many to read.
Titles I thought I had read

years before

were new, unopened.

I began crying out
In every way I knew
screaming
"I don't know
if I can finish this book
it's too hard!
I won't live through it!"

But time passed

thanks to the pills
every night
to ease the pain

Still I kept reading
always expecting
almost wanting
to die of sadness

because even though
every book was
different
than the rest
I'd gone my way
reading them all
the same.

Finally.
a month called March
turned on the calendar
and I was still alive
and my pain
subsided

five long months
that changed
my reading speed
the quality
of my prose

I still don't know
if I can finish this
book
but in knowing I want
to
I'm almost there

closing one book
with my right hand
lifting another
with my left
noticing each one,
each title is
different...
a peaceful, calming
scene.

October 12, 1985

Dear Mary,

My feelings range from sadness to relief to satisfaction as I write this last letter to you. Maybe some day I'll show you this pile of feelings. Or maybe you'll come across it some day in a bookstore, open it, and find yourself, and me, and all those others we love, plastered on the pages.

Whenever you get the chance to read this, I want to say thanks, for listening.

I love you,
Linda

Was It Always Like This?

Was it always like this?
Living each day
to its fullest
Living each day
to its last?

Did I always wake up
every morning
thinking
this may be my final say
I'll make sure I live it
in a way different
from the past.

What's different about me
 now?
I can bend each thing
that happens to me
 good or bad
 to fit my life.

The difference is loud
the difference is dear

it's my ability
to savor
expression.